IMMUNOLOGY AND IMMUNE SYSTEM DISORDERS

TECHNIQUES IN EPIDERMAL BIOLOGY

AN INTEGRATED APPROACH TO AUTOIMMUNE SKIN DISEASE

IMMUNOLOGY AND IMMUNE SYSTEM DISORDERS

Additional books in this series can be found on Nova's website under the Series tab.

Additional E-books in this series can be found on Nova's website under the E-books tab.

DERMATOLOGY - LABORATORY AND CLINICAL RESEARCH

Additional books in this series can be found on Nova's website under the Series tab.

Additional E-books in this series can be found on Nova's website under the E-books tab.

IMMUNOLOGY AND IMMUNE SYSTEM DISORDERS

TECHNIQUES IN EPIDERMAL BIOLOGY

AN INTEGRATED APPROACH TO AUTOIMMUNE SKIN DISEASE

NICOLA CIRILLO
EDITOR

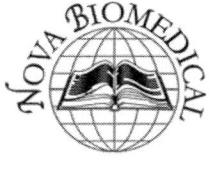

Nova Biomedical Books
New York

Copyright © 2012 by Nova Science Publishers, Inc.

All rights reserved. No part of this book may be reproduced, stored in a retrieval system or transmitted in any form or by any means: electronic, electrostatic, magnetic, tape, mechanical photocopying, recording or otherwise without the written permission of the Publisher.

For permission to use material from this book please contact us:
Telephone 631-231-7269; Fax 631-231-8175
Web Site: http://www.novapublishers.com

NOTICE TO THE READER

The Publisher has taken reasonable care in the preparation of this book, but makes no expressed or implied warranty of any kind and assumes no responsibility for any errors or omissions. No liability is assumed for incidental or consequential damages in connection with or arising out of information contained in this book. The Publisher shall not be liable for any special, consequential, or exemplary damages resulting, in whole or in part, from the readers' use of, or reliance upon, this material. Any parts of this book based on government reports are so indicated and copyright is claimed for those parts to the extent applicable to compilations of such works.

Independent verification should be sought for any data, advice or recommendations contained in this book. In addition, no responsibility is assumed by the publisher for any injury and/or damage to persons or property arising from any methods, products, instructions, ideas or otherwise contained in this publication.

This publication is designed to provide accurate and authoritative information with regard to the subject matter covered herein. It is sold with the clear understanding that the Publisher is not engaged in rendering legal or any other professional services. If legal or any other expert assistance is required, the services of a competent person should be sought. FROM A DECLARATION OF PARTICIPANTS JOINTLY ADOPTED BY A COMMITTEE OF THE AMERICAN BAR ASSOCIATION AND A COMMITTEE OF PUBLISHERS.

Additional color graphics may be available in the e-book version of this book.

Library of Congress Cataloging-in-Publication Data
Cirillo, Nicola, DDS.
  Techniques in epidermal biology : an integrated approach to autoimmune skin disease / Nicola Cirillo.
       p. ; cm.
  Includes bibliographical references and index.
  ISBN 978-1-61209-621-6 (softcover : alk. paper)
  1. Pemphigus--Pathophysiology. 2. Epidermolysis bullosa--Pathophysiology.
I. Title.
  [DNLM: 1. Pemphigus. 2. Acantholysis. WR 200]
  RL301.C57 2011
  616.5--dc22
                          2011003591

Published by Nova Science Publishers, Inc. † New York

To my family

Contents

Preface		vii
Chapter 1	Pathophysiology of the Epidermis: Lesson from Pemphigus	1
Chapter 2	Patients, Sera, and Experimental Models	21
Chapter 3	Optimization of the Experimental Procedures: Semi-Quantitative LCIF Microscopy, Cirillo's HSU Buffer, KAD Medium	37
Chapter 4	Study of Anti-Desmoglein Autoimmunity: Pemphigus Vulgaris as a Desmoglein-Remodeling Disease	49
Chapter 5	Role of Non-Desmoglein and Non-IgG Autoimmunity in PV	77
Chapter 6	Downstream Signaling Involved in Acantholysis: Part I: Changes in Cell Cycle and Protein Phosphorylation	95
Chapter 7	Downstream Signaling Involved in Acantholysis: Part II: Secretion of Proteinases and the "Specific Proteolysis Hypothesis" of Pemphigus	111
Chapter 8	Microarray Analysis of Diseased Tissues: Cell Adhesion Is Down-Regulated on the Gene Level in Pemphigus	123

Chapter 9	Pharmacological Block of Acantholysis: Towards Novel Therapies for the Treatment of Pemphigus	**139**
Acknowledgments		**153**
References		**155**
Index		**169**

Preface

The high-throughput techniques underlying a systems level analysis of biological organisms have emerged as powerful tools in the study of disease mechanisms. On the other hand, they require substantial funding and multidisciplinary skills. Therefore, basic biochemical and cell biology methods from molecular bioscience are still needed to address key biological questions. In the present book, a sequence of laboratory techniques and methods is presented, including cell culture, Western blotting, immunofluorescence, immunohistochemistry, zymography, ELISA, DNA microarrays. Tools are provided to implement the above techniques and reproduce experimental models of human disease. The authors used the autoimmune disease Pemphigus Vulgaris (PV) to model disruption of epidermal integrity and to study complex physiological networks involved in skin physiology. A progression from simple molecular bioscience principles to high-throughput methods are presented, which lead to a better understanding of disease pathophysiology and novel therapeutic modalities.

Chapter 1

Pathophysiology of the Epidermis: Lesson from Pemphigus

Epidermal autoimmune diseases such as Pemphigus provide an attractive model for studying complex physiological networks involved in regulating epidermal integrity. Pemphigus is a group of life-threatening autoimmune blistering diseases targeting skin and mucous membranes. Pemphigus vulgaris (PV) is the most common type of pemphigus and affects primarily the oral mucosa. It is characterised by disruption of cell adhesion among keratinocytes termed acantholysis.

To date, two main classes of autoantigens are thought to play a role in PV pathogenesis: of these, desmosomal cadherins (desmoglein 1 and 3) are the best characterized and considered as the most important. Additional antigens include the novel epithelial acetylcholine receptors ($\alpha 9$ and pemphaxin). Thus, acantholysis in pemphigus seems to result from a cooperative action of antibodies to different keratinocyte self-antigens, but the mechanisms by which the epithelial cleft occurs are not yet clearly understood.

In fact, the binding of PV autoantibodies to their targets generates a plethora of biological effects due, on one hand, to their direct interference with adhesive function and, on the other, to more complex events involving transduction of signals to the cell. These intracellular pathways could modify kinase and protease activity, leading to loss of cell-cell adhesion.

Introduction

Skin is the largest organ of the human body and acts as the major barrier against external environment. Epidermal autoimmune diseases provide an attractive model for studying complex physiological networks involved in regulating epidermal integrity. Circulating autoantibodies to normal constituents of keratinocyte surface molecules cause loss of adhesion in epidermal cells, blister formation and extensive skin wounding which can lead to a fatal outcome. The mode by which autoimmune sera orchestrate such life-threatening events and the experimental methods employed to investigate the underlying pathophysiological mechanisms are the focus of the present book..

Epidermal strength and integrity are provided by a class of specialized junctions called "anchoring junctions", comprised of a) adherens junctions that associate with actin microfilaments at cell-cell interfaces and b) desmosomes that anchor intermediate filaments (keratins) at sites of strong intercellular adhesion.

The most prominent organelles in epidermal tissue, desmosomes, provide strength to tissues which experience mechanical stress, such as epidermis and heart. Desmosomes are impaired in pemphigus, a potentially fatal blistering disease of the skin and mucous membranes characterized by the loss of intercellular adhesion of keratinocytes.

Pemphigus (from Greek pemphix, *pustule*) is a group chronic tissue-specific autoimmune blistering diseases targeting skin and mucous-membranes [1]. The common lesion of all types of pemphigus is the disruption on cell-cell adhesion among keratinocytes with subsequent intraepithelial splitting, or acantholysis.

Over the nineties, significant progress in understanding the nature of autoantibodies and cognate antigens has led to a novel classification of pemphigus subtypes [2] (table 1).

PV autoantibodies (PV IgG) are detected bound to the surface of lesional epidermis and circulating in the patients' serum [3-5]. PV IgG titres seem to correlate with the extent and the activity of PV as demonstrated by indirect immunofluorescence (IIF) titres as a measure of the pemphigus antibody levels [6, 7].

Table 1. Types of pemphigus and respective desmosomal autoantigens

Types	Autoantibodies	Target antigens
Classic pemphigus		
1. Pemphigus vulgaris (mucosal domynant type)	IgG	Dsg3 (130 kDa)
2. Pemphigus vulgaris (mucocutaneous type)	IgG	Dsg3 Dsg1 (160 kDa) Dsc3
3. Pemphigus foliaceus	IgG	Dsg1
Variant of classic pemphigus		
4. Herpetiform pemphigus	IgG	Dsg1 Dsg3
New pemphigus		
5. Paraneoplastic pemphigus	IgG	Dsg 3 Dsg 1 Plakins *
6. IgA pemphigus a. subcorneal pustular dermatosis (SPD) type	IgA	Desmocollin 1 (115/105 kDa)
b. intraepidermal neutrophilic type (IEN)	IgA	?
c. Pemphigus vulgaris (PV) type	IgA	Dsg3
d. Pemphigus foliaceus (PF)type	IgA	Dsg1

*Pectin (500 kDa), Desmoplakin I, II (250 kDa, 210 kDa), BPAG1 (230 kDa), Envoplakin (210 kDa), Periplakin (190 kDa), ? (170 kDa).

Pemphigus Vulgaris

The most common type of pemphigus, presents in middle-aged and genetically predisposed individuals with only oral lesions in one half to two thirds of patients, in contrast to pemphigus foliaceus in which mucous membrane involvement is usually absent.

Oral blisters are fragile and rupture readily, leaving erosions which are hard to heal. Mucosal dominant type of PV shows predominant oral erosions with limited skin involvement, which are no more than five or six erosions or blisters [2].

Among the array of keratinocyte self antigens immunoprecipitated by circulating PV IgG [8, 9], the best characterized is desmoglein (Dsg) 3, desmosomal glycoprotein which is critically involved in ensuring calcium-dependent intercellular adhesion among keratinocytes [10].

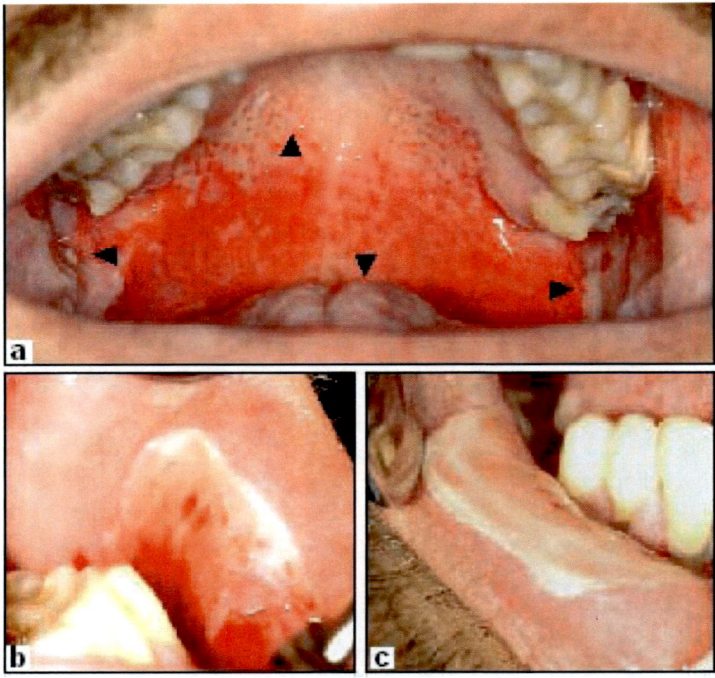

Figure 1. Involvement of the oral mucosa. Typical oral erosions with irregular margins covered by whitish pseudomembranes on tongue, buccal mucosa (bilaterally), and palate (a, arrowheads). In this patient, the lesions also affected mucosa of lips (b, c).

Indeed, mucosal PV associates with the presence of circulating IgG against linear and conformational epitopes of Dsg3. Subsequently, flaccid bullae may develop over several sites of the skin (trunk, scalp, flexures). The blistering is not always obvious, and often most lesions consist of crusted erosions. Skin involvement and disease progression correlate with the appearance of IgG against Dsg1, a cell adhesion protein strictly related to Dsg3 [11]. In general, the mucocutaneous type tends to be generalized and, therefore, more severe than the oral dominant type. Left untreated, the disease progresses with an almost always fatal outcome owing to uncontrolled fluid and protein loss or opportunistic infection.

Immunopathology of PV

The hallmark of histologic changes in pemphigus is the intra-epithelial cleft that results from cell-cell dyshesion (acantholysis) with formation of bullae containing isolated, round-shaped, acantholytic (or Tzanck) cells. The cleft is suprabasal in pemphigus vulgaris and vegetans, subcorneal in the pemphigus foliaceus subtypes. A mild to moderate inflammatory infiltrate may be seen in the upper dermis [1].

The epidermal antigen recognised by PV autoantibodies has been identified as a 130-kDa glycoprotein that is immunoprecipitated from keratinocyte extract as part of the "PV complex", which also includes the 85-kDa molecule plakoglobin [12, 13]. The cDNA encoding the PV antigen has been cloned and sequenced, identifying the antigen as desmoglein 3 (Dsg3), a desmosomal glycoprotein that belongs to the cadherin family of calcium-dependent cell adhesion molecules [10]. Dsg3 forms intercellular bridges by binding controlateral desmosomal halves in an homophylic and eterophylic manner (Figure 2) It seems that PVIgG recognises Dsg3 conformational epitopes formed by the N-terminal 161 amino acid, that are thought to contain sequences functionally critical for cadherin-mediated cell-cell adhesion [14-18]. However, about one-half to two-thirds of PV sera also contain antibodies against Dsg1 and some of these react with Dsg4, although this finding is a result of the cross-reactivity of a small subset of anti-Dsg1 autoantibodies [19]. Today, it is widely accepted that anti-Dsg1 autoantibodies in PV are pathogenic [11, 20]. Furthermore, some putative non-Dsg pemphigus antigens represent other adhesion molecules, such as plakoglobin [21], desmocollins [22], desmoplakin [23] and collagen XVII/BP180 [24]. Other pemphigus antigens include keratinocyte acetylcholine receptors (AChR) targeted by autoantibodies produced by pemphigus patients [25], annexins and the annexin-like molecule pemphaxin [26, 27].

Moreover, it seems that the phenomenon of acantholysis is related to a series of cytokines, such as IL-1α, TNF-α [28, 29], IL-6 [30] and IL-10 [31, 32], but these associations are not yet clear. Recently, a pivotal role in generating keratinocyte dyshesion has been suggested for apoptosis [33-35], but further studies to confirm this hypothesis are required.

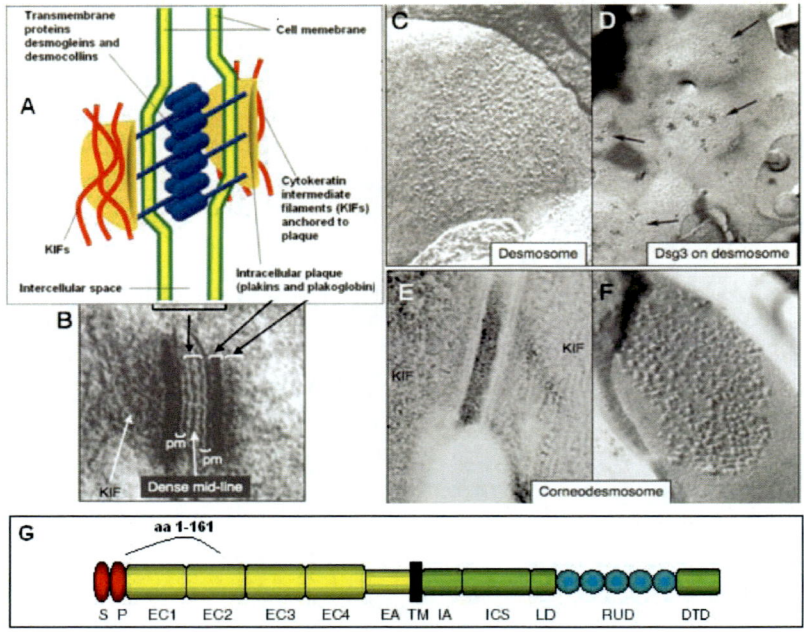

Figure 2. Scheme of molecular organization of desmosomal components (A) and thin section electron micrographs (B). Freeze-fracture electron (C) and immunoelectron micrographs (D) of desmosomes in keratinocytes before cornification. In the freeze-fracture immunoelectron micrograph, Dsg3 protein particles are decorated with anti-Dsg3 antibody (PV-IgG) with gold particles (D). Thin section (E) and freeze-fracture (F) electron micrographs of desmosomes of cornified keratinoctyes. (G) The structural organization of desmogleins. Dsg3, as a member of the cadherin superfamily is type I transmembrane protein and contains characteristic extracellular cadherin repeats (EC1-4) and a more variable fifth extracellular anchor domain (EA) close to the transmembrane domain (TM). Dsg3 structure includes an intracellular anchor domain (IA) and an intracellular cadherin-specific domain (ICS). The cytoplasmic domains of Dsg3 are extended by an intracellular proline-rich linker (LD or IPL), a repeating unit domain (RUD) and a C-terminal desmoglein-specific terminal domain (DTD).

Although the anti-desmoglein antibodies have been shown to cause the clinical and histologic lesions in pemphigus, the specific pathophysiological mechanism by which they do so remains controversial. Desmoglein compensation theory has suggested that PV IgG can cause direct inhibition of desmogleins' adhesive function through steric hindrance [18, 20]. Alternatively, or additionally, Dsg3 can act as a receptor by triggering complex intracellular events, including changes in intracellular calcium concentration, PKC and p38 MAPK activation, apoptosis, transcriptional regulation and proteinase activity, all causing desmosome disassembly [36-41]. Furthermore, binding of autoantibodies to Dsg3 could modulate its own synthesis, leading to the formation of aberrant desmosomes lacking Dsg3 both *in vitro* [42] and *in vivo* [43].

In the last years, beside these theories sharing the desmoglein autoimmunity, the attention of many investigators was pointed towards the pathophysiological role of non-desmoglein targets in pemphigus vulgaris, represented by acetylcholine receptors α9 and pemphaxin [25, 27] members of the cholinergic axis, in which the "cytotransmitter" acetylcholine (ACh) is involved in the control of the keratinocyte-keratinocyte adhesion.

Plasminogen Activation Hypothesis

Cellular plasminogen activators are secreted serine proteases which convert the zymogen plasminogen to active trypsin-like proteinase plasmin. In the epidermis, this mechanism serves to generate plasmin activity in the pericellular space, thus regulating cell adhesion and migration [44].

One of the first hypotheses that tried to clarify PV pathogenesis suggested blister formation being mediated by release of nonlysosomal proteases secondary to antibody binding [45]. Indeed, Schiltz et al. showed that when suspensions of primary human epidermal cells were incubated with pemphigus IgG, a rapid solubilisation of insoluble cellular material occurred and the cells were eventually killed. It was suggested that this phenomenon was caused by a nonlysosomal proteolytic enzyme (because it was maximally active at pH 6.5), which was synthesised, released or activated by the epidermal cell. This "pemphigus acantholysis factor" (PAF) was expressed in human epidermal cells following their interaction with pemphigus antibody and caused epidermal acantholysis in fresh skin explants [45]. Plasmin appeared to be the active enzyme in producing acantholysis [46]. This view has been supported by several observations (table 2). Thus, a possible signalling pathway mediating PV-IgG induced cell-cell detachment may be the following: PV-IgG induces aberrant signal transduction, which mediates Dsg3 phosphorylation and leads to its dissociation from plakoglobin. This may impair desmosome formation from the inside of the cell by leading to depletion of Dsg3 from desmosomes and by inducing uPAR transcription PG-mediated. PV-IgG also induces PKC signalling, which is involved in uPA secretion and uPAR expression on the cell surface, leading to activation of plasmin; this signal may then mediate the dissociation of pre-existing desmosomes from the outside of the cell. These two different PV-IgG-activated signaling pathways could be responsible for the mechanism of generation of acantholysis in PV (Figure 3).

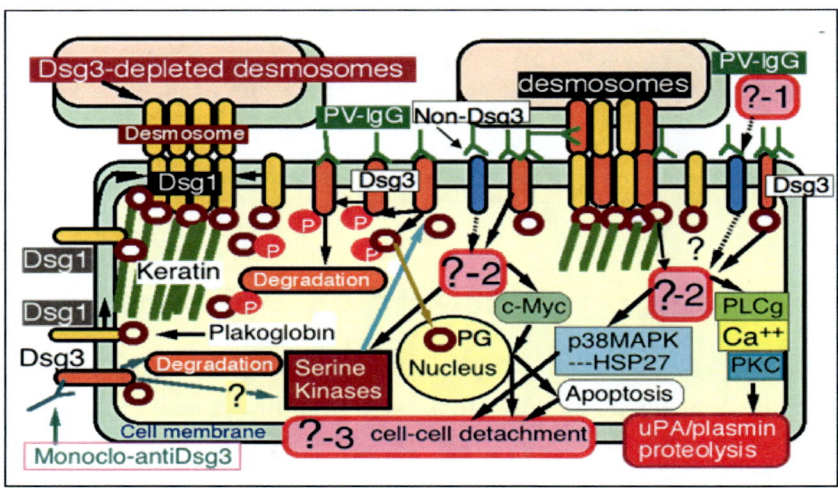

Figure 3. Schematic model illustrating plausible PV-IgG-induced cellular events that may be linked activation of plasminogen [96]. Question 1 (?-1) indicates PV-IgG autoantibodies binding to antigens and receptors other than Dsg3. Question 2 (?-2) indicates a variety of unknown signaling cascades, that mediate to serine kinase to phosphorylate Dsg3, PLC/ Ca++/PKC pathway linked to uPA/uPA activation, p38MAPK and apoptosis pathways. It has been shown that pathogenic monoclonal anti-Dsg3 antibodies causes Dsg3 degradation leading to formation of Dsg3-depleted desmosomes (illustrated at the left part of the figure). Although Dsg3-depletion from desmosome may be implicated to reduce the adhesive mechanical strength and uPA/plasmin proteolysis to be implicated to digest desmosomes at outside of the cell, possible mechanisms underling how to link p38MAPK and apoptosis signaling to cause cell-cell detachment are unknown (question 3: ?-3). From: Kitajima Y, Aoyama Y. In: Cirillo N, Ed. 2009. Pathophysiology of the desmosome. Research Signpost. Kerala.

Why plasminogen hypothesis is an untenable model of pathogenesis. The theory tracing acantholysis back to serum proteinases activity is that had more credibility in the past. Today, the central role of plasmin in inducing cell-cell detachment is difficult to sustain. The reasons for that are well argumented in a recent review by the Author, and may be summarized as follows:

The uPAR is expressed by keratinocytes during re-epithelialisation of skin wounds. The plasminogen activation system plays a prominent role in cell migration by regulating the pericellular proteolytic events required to release cell to cell adhesion [47]. Thus, the acantholytic cleft could be taken as representing an epithelial wound and the overregulation of uPA/uPAR system could similarly be taken as representing the initial step by keratinocytes to attempt to repair the damage.

Serum is a potent stimulator of PA activity. In lesional epidermis from patients with a variety of cutaneous diseases, including pemphigus vulgaris, tPA is selectively elevated in the suprabasal layers and becomes the predominant PA activity. Since serum is a potent stimulator of tPA synthesis [48], plasminogen activation may represent an event following epithelial damage, perhaps after plasma infiltration into lesional epidermis (as classically occurs in pemphigus, with the formation of aphlegmasic blister) and provide an explanation for the "low acantholysis" typical of PV.

PV and PF antibodies are pathogenic in plasminogen activator knockout mice. The importance of plasminogen activator in blister formation pathogenesis during PV has been checked using PA knockout mice [49]. After passive transfer of PF and PV IgG these mice blistered to the same degree as the single knockout and the control mice, and histology indicated blisters at the expected level of the epidermis. These data demonstrate that PA is not necessary for pemphigus IgG-mediated acantholysis in mouse.

Direct Steric Hindrance of Cell-Cell Adhesion and Desmoglein Compensation Theory

Earlier studies on *in vitro* models of PV suggested that cell-cell detachment was likely to occur as a consequence of the autoantibody binding to keratinocyte surface proteins and their internalization [50]. Accordingly, Jones hypothesized that acantholysis was generated from the direct interference of PV-IgG with the normal desmosomal functions [51]. Years later, with the advent of modern technologies, the study on the expression pattern of PV antigens Dsg1 and Dsg3 within the epidermis, together with the clinical, pathological and laboratoristic correlations of the disease, altogether led to the well known "desmoglein compensation" theory [2, 20]. Subsequent studies postulated that PV IgG could directly interfere with the adhesion function of desmogleins by steric hindrance [18, 19]. These findings served as a further validation of the compensation hypothesis, although it should be emphasized that the two concepts are not necessarily overlapping. Today this theory is accepted by most of the authors. The main findings in support to the desmoglein compensation theory are summarized in table 2.

Desmogleins spatial expression as an explanation the localization of acantholysis in PV patients' cutaneus and mucous epithelia. It has been suggested that the distribution and expression levels of Dsg1 and Dsg3 might account for the characteristic distribution and localisation of the blisters in PV and PF patients [20]. It is known that Dsg3 is expressed throughout the oral mucosa, especially in the upper two-thirds, whereas in the epidermis it is expressed only in the basal and immediate suprabasal layer. Conversely, Dsg1 is expressed throughout the epidermis and oral mucosa, but more intensely in the subcorneal layer, and very weakly in the deep epidermis [52].

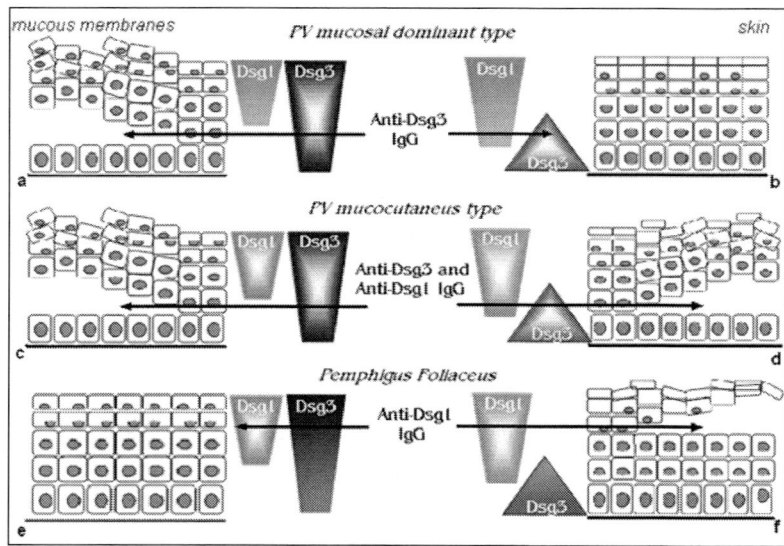

Figure 4. Schematic representation of the desmoglein compensation hypothesis. This theory established strict correlation between clinical phenotype and anti-desmoglein autoantibody profile. See text for details.

It has been proven that the clinical phenotype of the pemphigus is defined by the anti-desmoglein autoantibody profile [53]. So, patients with pemphigus have anti-Dsg1 and/or anti-Dsg3 IgG autoantibodies but no anti-Dsg2 autoantibodies. Some patients with PV have only anti-Dsg3 IgG, whereas other PV patients have both anti-Dsg3 and anti-Dsg1 IgG, as found by immunoprecipitation and by immunofluorescence of Dsg1 transfected cells.

Patients with PF have only anti-Dsg1 IgG as observed by immunoprecipitation and immunoadsorption assay with recombinant Dsg1 [53, 54].

Based on the above findings and speculation that Dsg1 and Dsg3 compensate their adhesive function when they are coexpressed on the same cell, the localisation of blister formation in pemphigus can be explained very well. In fact, PF anti-Dsg1 IgG causes blisters in the superficial layers of the epidermis but not in the deep epidermis or mucosa, where the expression of Dsg3 compensates for the antibody-induced functional loss of Dsg1. Similarly, in mucosal PV, anti-Dsg3 IgG causes acantholysis in the deepest layer of the mucous membranes where Dsg1 expression is minimal [55]. Moreover, in mucocutaneous PV both anti-Dsg1 and anti-Dsg3 antibodies are required for pathogenicity, so that also in the epidermis "low acantholysis" occurs (Figure 4). The cell-cell adhesion between the basal and the immediate suprabasal layers might be weaker than the other parts of the epidermis because there are fewer desmosomes. In addition, the lower part of the epidermis might have better access for autoantibodies which penetrate from the dermis. That may explain why the splits become suprabasilar in mucocutaneous PV [2].

Take together, these studies show that in PV Dsg3 and Dsg1 can compensate for one another in maintaining keratinocyte adhesion and, at the same time, suggest that pemphigus autoantibodies can directly interfere with cell adhesion by steric hindrance (table 1). This Dsg compensation hypothesis is incompatible with the protease theory of blister formation. In fact, if proteases were the major cause of the acantholytic cleft in pemphigus, then binding of autoantibodies to either Dsg1 or Dsg3 would cause protease release and blister formation and prevent functional compensation of one by the other.

Antibody-mediated direct steric hindrance and desmoglein compensation cannot completely explain the mechanisms of acantholysis pemphigus. In the article by Sergei Grando and colleagues " Pemphigus: an unfolding story", the Authors refused the desmoglein compensation theory by raising a series of questions. (i) Why would PV patients harbouring both Dsg1 and Dsg3 antibodies develop only suprabasilar rather than suprabasilar and subcorneal blisters? (ii) Why does Dsg1 antibody not cause a granular layer split in PV? (iii) Why do some people who have circulating anti-Dsg1 and/or Dsg3 antibodies not manifest pemphigus? [56].

A number of observations in fact question the exclusive role of Dsgs in pemphigus. The flaws of desmoglein compensation theory have been recently reviewed by us [57] and are summarized below:

Inconsistencies between clinical phenotype and antibodies profile. The desmoglein compensation hypothesis foresees an exact correlation between clinical/histological manifestations and the autoantibody profile, establishing clearly distinguishable classic pemphigus types.

There are a number of studies showing pemphigus features with clinical shifting between pemphigus foliaceus (PF) and pemphigus vulgaris (PV) and vice versa. However, according to this theory is very difficult to explain the presence of both Dsg1 and Dsg3 antibodies in cases of PF that show the typical subcorneal acantholysis without oral manifestations [58]. We too have recently reported a patient with PV dysplayng skin lesions resembling pemphigus erythematosus [59].

Almost 50% of first-degree relatives of PV patients present circulating PV- IgG. It is accepted that between 40% and 71% of immediate relatives of pemphigus patients have been found to be carriers of low-titres of PV autoantibodies even if they have no clinical manifestation [60]. One possible explanation may relie in the amount of pathogenic PV-IgG and/or in the different degree of pathogenicity due to recognition of functionally nonessential epitopes. The different degree of pathogenicity can be due also to the different prevalence of the IgG-isoform, i.e. IgG4 vs. IgG1 subtype [60-63].

Dsg1 and Dsg3 antibodies are not unique to pemphigus. Patients with silicosis without bullous disease may develop antibodies to Dsg1 and/or to Dsg3 [64]. Moreover, sera from 80% of subjects with periodontitis showed increased reactions of IgG with Dsg (165, 130 and 115kDa) compared with unaffected controls [56]. Accordingly, antidesmosomal antibodies may be considered as a normal part of the immune repertoire. It is interesting that recently this has been detected in 55% of normal subjects from Limao Verde, an endemic area for Fogo Selvagem [65, 66].

PV-IgG induce neither the intercellular loss adhesion nor the desmosome disassembly in PG -/- cell-culture. As described previously, keratinocyte cultures from plakoglobin knockout (PG -/-) mice embryos are not responsive to PV-IgG stimulation, which means that the simple binding of PV-IgG to Dsg3 is not sufficient to induce KIF retraction and acantholysis *in vitro* [67].

Dsg1 and Dsg3 could be not essential for keratinocytes adhesion. It has been known that the stability of desmosomal junctions also relies on Dsg2 and desmocollins [68] and that the expression of Dsg1 compensates for genetic loss of Dsg3-mediated adhesion [69].

Moreover Dsg1 and Dsg3 are not sufficient to support cell-cell adhesion when expressed in nonadhesive fibroblast-like cells and, however, for the most part, authors have not been able to convincingly demonstrate the adhesive capacity of the Dsg *in vitro* [70-72]. The inactivation of the Dsg3 gene or depletion of Dsg3 from keratinocytes within the epidermis of experimental animals or in cultured monolayers fails to induce gross skin blistering or disrupt desmosomes respectively [43, 73]. These data question the role of the Dsgs in cell-cell adhesion.

Acetylcholine Receptors and the "Multiple Hit" Hypothesis

In the last lustre, there have been many studies showing that the autoimmunty in pemphigus is not only limited to anti-Dsg antibodies: to date, a catalogue of self antigens, demonstrated by various authors and detection techniques to react uniquely with PV-IgG, includes approximately 20 molecules with different relative molecular masses, namely: 12, 18, 33, 47, 50, 52, 55, 59, 66, 67, 68, 75, 78, 80, 85, 102, 105, 160, 180, 185/190 and 210 kDa [74]. The number of detectable target molecules varies from patient to patient and depends on the sensitivity of the detection technique, i.e., immunoblotting versus immunoprecipitation. Hypothetically, some of these bands may represent degradation products of pemphigus antigens having higher native molecular weights, but the studies demonstrating that molecules different from Dsg1 and Dsg3 represent the autoantigens of the PV-IgG are becoming numerous. It is known that non-Dsg3/non-Dsg1 PV-IgG induce PV-like lesions in neonatal mice; moreover, rDsg3-Ig absorb non-Dsg3 antibodies that are pathogenic in Dsg3-null mice [8]. These data strongly suggest that autoantibodies other than anti-Dsg1 and anti-Dsg3 are involved in PV autoimmunity: thus, target antigens are not restricted to desmoglein. Some of these antigens have been identified a epidermal acetylcholine receptors (AChR). Indeed, human epidermal keratinocytes are members of a non-neuronal signalling network mediating intercellular communication in the skin in which the cytotransmitter acetylcholine (ACh) acts as a local hormone, or a cytokine. Non-neuronal ACh is responsible for dramatic effects on the keratinocytes' proliferation, migration and differentiation, more than for intercellular adhesion and for other sublayers [75, 76]. In several cell types, activation of AChRs affects signalling pathways regulating the expression and/or function of adhesion molecules [77, 78] as well as the protein phosphorylation status [79, 80]. Regarding the role of the epithelial cholinergic system in PV, it has been reported that (reviewed in ref. 81): ***a.*** approximately 85% of pemphigus patients develop antibodies against keratinocyte AChR ***b.***

acantholytic activity of the PV-IgG feigns pharmacologic effects on the keratinocytes' shape and binding-adhesive property similar to cholinergic antagonists c. acantholyitic antibodies are able to recognise another two receptorial molecules other than Dsg: 1) the α9 acetylcholine receptor, a 50 kDa homopentamer which regulates the adhesion in the epithelial cells [25] and 2) pemphaxin, a 75 kDa novel annexin (also known annexin 31 or ANXA9) that can act as an acetylcholine receptor [27]. The demonstration that cholinomimetics drugs such as carbachol and pyridostigmine bromide can improve, and in some cases prevent acantohlysis *in vivo* [82], suggests that ACh and its receptors could be involved in the pathogenesis of acantholysis, giving us new prospects for the nonhormonal treatment of pemphigus patients [83].

The Multiple Hit hypothesis of pemphigus. The desmoglein theory of PV pathogenesis is based on the assumption that antibodies against Dsg1/Dsg3 should by itself be able to cause pemphigus. Nevertheless, autoantibodies absorbed with extracellular epitope of Dsg3 are not capable to induce gross blisters in the skin of neonatal mice, whereas the eluant from the chimeric baculoprotein by itself did produce blisters [15].

Thus, acantholysis in pemphigus seems to result from a cooperative action of antibodies to different keratinocyte self-antigens, including both regulatory molecules, such as AChRs, and structural molecules, such as desmosomal cadherins.

Most recently, a 130kD antigen other than Dsg3, has been immunoprecipitated with PV-IgG from peripheral blood mononuclear cells [9]. These findings have fostered an alternative concept of pathophysiologic relevance of non-desmoglein targets in PV known as "multiple hit" hypothesis (Figure 5).

This hypothesis states that Dsg3 is only one among different antigens recognized by PV sera, each of which contributes in a unique way to a loss of cell adhesion and blister formation in PV. Furthermore, it is not excluded that PV-IgG action toward AChRs could indirectly influence the mechanisms of cell adhesion.

In fact, it is known that α9 receptor stimulation induces phosphorilation of membrane-associated 120 and 220 kDa proteins which may be represented by adhesion molecules such as E-cadherin and desmoplakin II [25, 84].

Moreover, the cholinergic agonist carbachol, which can prevent and reverse pemphigus IgG-induced acantholysis *in vitro*, seems to activate cell adhesive function by stimulating Dsg1/3 expression and E-cadherin activity [77, 78].

Taken together, these data suggest that acantholysis is, at least partially, the result of an IgG antagonism against AChR and that cell adhesion cholinergic control coupled with ACh-receptor transduction pathways can be restored by an excess of agonists which protect receptorial sites from antibody binding through a competitive inhibition mechanism.

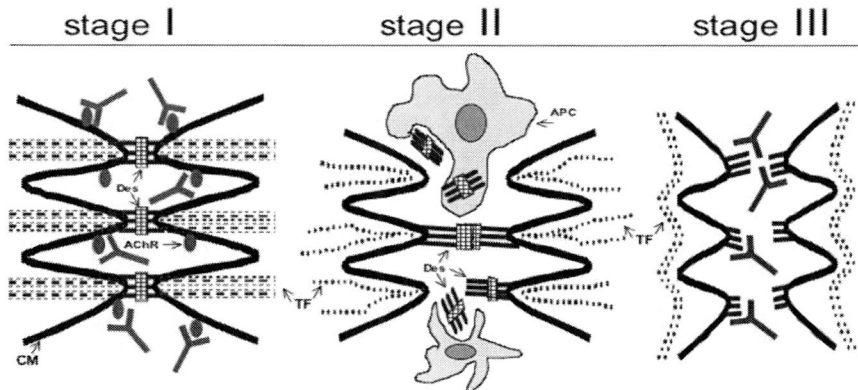

Figure 5. Hypothetical scheme of the time course events leading to acantholysis in pemphigus. In stage I, antibodies to acetylcholine receptors (AChR) block ACh signaling that maintains polygonal cell shape and intercellular adhesion. This increases phosphorylation of adhesion molecules with their subsequent dissociation from the adhesion units, and also initiates programmed cell death via apoptotic and/or oncotic pathways. In stage II, the cytoskeleton collapses and keratinocytes shrink, which is accompanied by sloughing of the cell membrane pieces containing desmosomal cadherins, which elicits autoimmune response to the desmoglein antigens. In stage III, anti-desmoglein antibodies bind to their targets on the cell membrane of KCs thus precluding formation of new intercellular junctions. APC, antigen-presenting cell; CM, cell membrane; Des, desmosome; TF, tonofilaments.

It is worth of note that $Ca^{2}+$-mediated actin polymerisation is the main driving force for the realisation of cell-cell attachment and that desmosome assembly is a passive process verifying after stable intercellular contacts are done [85]. These findings confirm the importance of the cholinergic axis, involved in structurating actin cytoskeleton and adherent junction, in the pathogenesis of PV-IgG-induced cell detachment.

In summary, this multiple hit hypothesis proposes that acantholysis in pemphigus is mediated by at least two complementary pathogenic pathways, namely 1) anticholinergic receptor antibodies that weaken intercellular adhesions between keratinocytes via inactivation of the cholinergic receptor-mediated physiologic control of cadherin (Dsg) expression and/or function and causes dyshesion, cell detachment and rounding up, or acantholysis and 2) antibodies to adhesion molecules that prevent formation of new desmosomes in acantholytic keratinocytes by blocking the extracellular domains of desmosomal cadherins that mediate homo- and heterophilic adhesion (Figure 5). Although exciting, this model needs to be confirmed by more exhaustive evidences in this field.

Intracellular Signaling in Acantholysis and Related Theories on Pemphigus Blistering

Induction of acantholysis is an active process that appears to be more complex than the simple interaction of antibodies with adhesion molecules. Cell surface-bound pemphigus IgG causes phosphatidylcholine-specific phospholipase C (PC-PLC) activation, an increase in inositol 1,4,5-trisphosphate (IP3) and diacylglycerol (DAG) production, and protein kinase C (PKC) activity [36, 37]; furthermore, there is an increase in intracellular calcium concentration, which appears to result from IP3-mediated release of intracellular stores [86]. Dsg3 is phosphorylated by a kinase other than PKC and appears to dissociate from plakoglobin (see below); this dissociation may explain the ability of PV sera to deplete Dsg3 from desmosomes [42, 43]. Recently, a crucial role in PV blistering has been demonstrated for p38 MAPK, c-myc, and RhoA [87-89]. It is also of interest the study on the ability of PV IgG and/or serum factors such as FasL in inducing keratinocyte apoptosis. The complex intracellular pathways triggered by PV-IgG are reviewed in figure 6.

The Keratinocyte Death Hypothesis and Apoptolysis

The "Keratinocyte Death" hypothesis derives from the "Multiple Hit" hypothesis but merits its own place in the discussion. The striking resemblance of apoptotic and acantholytic keratinocytes has raised the question of how PV IgG affected keratinocytes die. Surprisingly, not only the keratinocytes that have lost their contacts die by apoptosis, but pemphigus keratinocytes that still have functional desmosomes and appear unaltered in perilesional skin and in cell culture feature activation of the extrinsic apoptotic pathway involving caspases 3 and 8 [35].

Table 2. Experimental evidence on potential mechanisms involved in acantholysis

uPA/uPAR system

- Plasminogen activator system is altered in pemphigus vulgaris
- Pemphigus IgG induces expression of uPA and uPAR in vitro
- Anti-uPA and anti-uPAR antibody inhibit acantholysis
- Acantholysis is blocked by uPA inhibitors
- Proteinase inhibitors could prevent acantholysis
- Pemphigus IgG activates PKC, involved in uPA and uPAR expression
- Plakoglobin could promote uPAR expression

Direct steric hindrance

- PV-IgG recognises Dsg3 conformational epitopes containing sequences functionally crucial for cadherin-mediated cell-cell adhesion
- Desmogleins expression pattern and antibody profile correlate with sites of blister formation
- PV patients with skin lesions also have anti-Dsg1 IgG
- In mice, both anti-Dsg3 and anti-Dsg1 IgG are necessary to induce skin blisters formation
- DSG3-gene inactivation in mice produces lesions similar those seen in the (mucous) PV-patients
- Dsg3 forced expression prevents blister formation in mice injected with anti-Dsg1 autoantibodies

Nondesmoglein targets and AChR-9

- The self antigens reacting uniquely with PV-IgG include approximately 20 molecules
- Non-Dsg1 and non-Dsg3 serum antibodies from patients with pemphigus vulgaris are pathogenic
- rDsg3 can absorb non-Dsg3 antibodies that are pathogenic in Dsg3-null mice
- Acetylcholine α9 receptor is targeted by pemphigus vulgaris antibodies
- Pemphigus vulgaris antibody identifies pemphaxin
- Cholinomimetic drugs exhibit anti-acantholytic activity
- Cholinergic antagonists induce in-vitro acantholysis
- 85% of pemphigus patients develop antibodies against keratinocyte AChR
- Epithelial acetylcholine receptors regulate cell adhesion

In contrast, anticholinergic substances like atropine, mecamylamine and strychnine seem to induce apoptosis and acantholysis in organotypic epidermis equivalent via a caspase-8 independent intrinsic pathway [90]. In addition to caspase dependent apoptosis, calpain dependent oncosis (cell swelling by loss of volume control) seems to be stimulated in certain PV patients [91].

Both processes together are suspected to be responsible for the morphology of acantholytic cells (small apoptotic nucleus and clear swollen cytoplasm). Calpains are involved in the cleavage of adhesion molecules such as cadherins and have been shown to play a critical role in oncosis by increasing plasma membrane permeability [92]. Calpain inhibitors, just like caspase inhibitors, are capable of inhibiting PVIgG induced acantholysis in newborn mice [91].

In addition, PV IgG induces a significant increase in the RNA level of caspases 3 and 8 already after 12 h exposure of keratinocytes and at the protein level after 24 h exposure. In contrast, the protein levels of the apoptosis inhibitor protein FLIP-1 was downregulated. Perhaps, apoptosis of keratinocytes leads to a specific cleavage of desmosomal cadherins by caspases followed by release of desmosomal cadherins from the cell surface by a metalloproteinase activity. Thus, acantholysis in pemphigus is an active process resulting from the intracellular signaling of separate yet complementary pathways, i.e. apoptosis and oncosis triggered by IgG binding to the keratinocyte membrane antigens in a receptor–ligand fashion [91].

Additionally, in pemphigus receptor-mediated cell death seems to be induced by the activation of membrane FasR through the binding to its ligand (FasL). Indeed, FasL levels are markedly increased in sera from pemphigus patients, which have been demonstrated to trigger apoptosis through the activation of caspase 8. However, recent works have reported that both apoptotic pathways, namely the extrinsic or death receptor-mediated, and the intrinsic, mitochondria-dependent, could be involved in pemphigus-associated cell death [93]. The finding that caspase 3 and matrix metalloproteinase 9 [94] directly cleaves Dsg3 and other desmosomal proteins, thereby causing apoptotic disruption of desmosomes, further suggests a strict correlation between loss of keratinocyte adhesion and apoptosis.

To emphasize the fact that structural damage and death of keratinocytes in PV are mediated by the same set of enzymes, Grando and collaborators introduced the new term "**apoptolysis**" [158]. This term distinguishes the unique mechanism of autoantibody-induced keratinocyte damage in PV from other known forms of cell death.

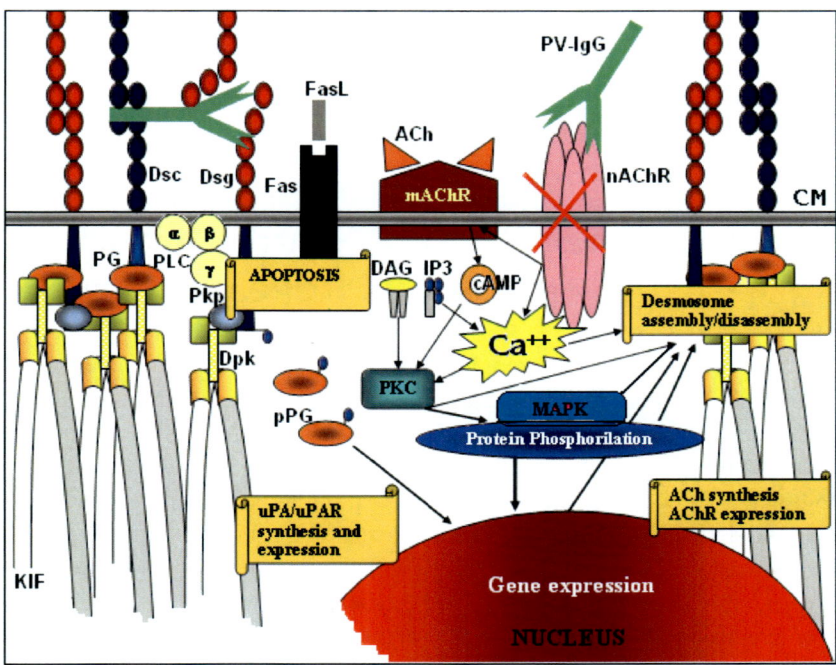

Figure 6. Intracellular pathways triggered by pemphigus serum in keratinocytes involve receptorial and non-receptorial signaling (see text for details). Modified from Lanza et al., 2006 [19].

The Basal Cell Shrinkage Hypothesis

The hypothesis proposed by Grando and Bystryn is that the binding of PV antibodies to keratinocytes triggers signaling and intracellular events that collapse the cytoskeletal structure of basal keratinocytes with consequent shrinkage of these cells [95]. Shrinking basal cells pull away from suprabasal cells (resulting in suprabasal acantholysis) and from each other (resulting in the "tombstone" appearance of basal cells). This explanation differs fundamentally from the current explanation for acantholysis, which argues the opposite - that acantholysis occurs because desmosomes lose their adhesive properties. This difference is critical to develop better ways of treating pemphigus, as discussed below. Authors further propose that acantholysis is limited to basal cells in PV because these cells shrink more than suprabasal keratinocytes when they interact with pemphigus antibodies. This could occur because basal cells are less rigid and shrink more readily than suprabasal keratinocytes when their cytoskeleton is altered, because their cytoskeletal structure is altered to a greater extent by the signaling event, or because different signaling events are triggered in basal cells.

Novel Concepts and Future Directions in Pemphigus Research

Over the last decade, pemphigus has evolved from the notion of a well-characterized autoimmune disease against a single adhesion molecule to that of a complex condition whose pathogenesis still remains to be fully elucidated. This apparent involution reflects the incongruence of a previously accepted dogmatic view of pemphigus as a paradigm of autoimmunity against desmoglein (Dsg) molecules. The discovery that autoimmunity in pemphigus was not restricted to Dsg1/3 shook scientists out of their torpor due to a belief that pemphigus was a "finished" disease [159]. Most important, the unconventional explanations for PV pathogenesis have given new lymph not only to the understanding of disease pathophysiology but, also, to our hopes for novel and more specific therapeutic modalities.

The fundamental myths that have been hampered pemphigus research toward development of a safe and efficient treatment are that: 1) the epidermal integrity is mediated exclusively by Dsg 1/3; 2) acantholysis is PV and PF is caused by steric hindrance of Dsg1/3; 3) clinical and histological features of autoimmune pemphigus can be reproduced solely by Dsg1/3 antibodies; 4) an interplay between Dsg1/3 antibodies determines the clinical phenotype; 5) the titers of Dsg1/3 antibodies correlate closely with the severely of disease; 6) the sera of pemphigus patients contain autoantibodies only to the Dsg 1/3 targets; and 7) CH treat pemphigus patients exclusively by inhibiting autoantibody production. As we have discussed above, recent advances of knowledge on pemphigus scrutinize old dogmas, resolve controversies and open novel perspectives for treatment. Further progress in understanding the molecular mechanisms mediating autoantibody production and apoptolysis in pemphigus should improve our understanding of disease pathogenesis and facilitate development of steroid free treatment of patients.

Chapter 2

Patients, Sera, and Experimental Models

Administration of IgG fractions or anti-Dsg3 IgG purified from sera of patients with pemphigus vulgaris (PV) is widely used to reproduce the disease both *in vitro* and *in vivo*. However, we have demonstrated that serum factors other than IgG can also participate to PV acantholysis, thus arising important methodological issues.

Indeed, the use of PV IgG or monoclonal anti-Dsg3 antibodies to experimentally reproduce the disease appears now inadequate, as it does not take into account the role of non-IgG factors. The use of whole sera for reproducing pemphigus-like lesions could help to overcome this methodological flaw.

However, the actual pathogenicity of whole sera in inducing clinical, histological and cytological changes typical of PV has not been systematically tested so far. Here, we addressed these questions by establishing experimental models of PV through the use of whole sera taken from patients with active disease.

Results showed that both human keratinocyte monolayers and mouse skin organ cultures responded to serum exposure by exhibiting the classical *in vitro* features of PV.

Furthermore, concentrated whole PV serum was able to reproduce PV-like lesions *in vivo* in neonatal mice. Thus, PV sera were able to induce clinical, histological and cytological changes typical of PV.

These data will enable us to utilize PV sera to model the disease without leaving serum factors other than IgG out of consideration.

Introduction

The immunopathogenesis of pemphigus vulgaris (PV) is not an "on-off" phenomenon. Rupture of the physiologic equilibrium leading to blister formation depends on autoantibody titers [7], intrinsic pathogenicity of the circulating autoantibody itself [17,18], patients' genetic background [96,97] and, possibly, ability of the host in maintaining tissue homeostasis [98]. It has been reported that more than one half of the immediate relatives of pemphigus patients are carriers of low-titres PV autoantibodies in absence of clinical manifestations [60]. Similarly, PV patients in clinical remission may show anti-intercellular substance (ICS) and anti-Dsg3 circulating autoantibodies, but it is well-known that no one utilizes these sera for its experiments. Furthermore, patients with silicosis and periodontitis without bullous disease may develop antibodies to Dsg1 and/or to Dsg3 [64]. Thus, the presence of circulating anti-ICS or anti-Dsg3 antibodies does not strictly correspond to the appearance of clinical manifestations. However, a critical discussion on the above concerns is now present in the literature [57].

Although a critical role for desmoglein (Dsg) 3 and Dsg1 targeting autoantibodies in PV seems undeniable, in recent years PV pathogenesis has been undergoing major revision, mostly because it has become clear that induction of cell-cell detachment is an active process that appears to be more complex than the unique interaction of such antibodies with adhesion molecules [8,57]. In addition, autoimmunity in pemphigus seems to be not just restricted to desmogleins; indeed, compelling evidence now attests to the role of IgG against keratinocyte cholinergic receptors in the disruption of cell-cell contacts leading keratinocytes to separate from one another [81]. Furthermore, pemphigus acantholysis is related to a series of cytokines, such as IL-1α, TNF-α [28,29], IL-6 [30] and IL-10 [31,32]. Although these molecules are unlikely to be pathogenic alone, they could be critical in regulating the delicate equilibrium that ensure the maintenance of cell adhesion. That is, these factors could participate as "supporting actors" in inducing blistering of PV patients' epidermis. Hence, a question raises: what should we use to experimentally reproduce the disease?

So far, the answers have been multiple. Total IgG from PV patients (PV IgG), polyclonal anti-Dsg3 antibody purified from patients' sera, and monoclonal anti-Dsg3 and/or anti-Dsg1 antibody, all have been used for establishing both *in vitro* and *in vivo* models of pemphigus [98,99]. However, before complicated techniques required for purification of antibodies were carried out, early studies on pemphigus were conducted by exposing human skin organ cultures to whole PV sera [100].

On these premises, in the present paper we attempted to establish *in vitro* – on both keratinocyte monolayers and skin organ cultures – and *in vivo* models of pemphigus vulgaris by using whole PV sera from patients with active disease.

Materials and Methods

Patients

Four patients with active PV (n=4, named PV1-4) who were not under corticosteroid therapy at the time of serum collection, and three volunteers without any skin disease (n=3, controls) have been enrolled for the study. The declaration of Helsinki protocols were followed and scientific committee of Center on Craniofacial Malformations - Regione Campania approved the study. Informed consent was obtained from all participants.

Diagnosis was established on the basis of results of both clinical and histological examinations, as detailed in Results section. The presence of autoantibodies was determined by both indirect immunofluorescence using monkey oesophagus as substrate (values above 1:80 of circulating anti-ICS antibodies were considered as positive) and Western blot analysis against Dsg3 and Dsg1. Patients with PV were classified as having mucosal type and mucocutaneous type based on clinical features and autoantibody profile assessed by ELISA against Dsg1 and Dsg3; an index value above 20.0 was considered to be positive [2]. All sera were heated to 56°C for 30 min to inactivate complement and then stored at -80°C.

Purification of Total IgG Fractions and Anti-Dsg3-L IgG

Sera of PV patients and healthy donors were collected. Anti-Dsg3-L antibodies from PV sera were purified in accordance with the procedure for immunoaffinity antibody purification [101]. Briefly, HaCaT detergent extracts were immunoprecipitated with the 5H10 antibody (Santa Cruz Biotecnology, Santa Cruz, CA) and the resulting antibody-antigen complexes were denatured and resolved by 8% SDS-polyacrylamide gel electrophoresis (PAGE). Filters were blocked with 5% nonfat milk in TBS-T (w/v) after which approximately

5-mm-wide horizontal strips carrying the 130-140 kDa Dsg3 were cut out from the immunoblotting membrane and incubated overnight with PV serum at 4°C. The IgG fractions bound to linear epitopes of Dsg3 were then eluted by a 20 mM sodium citrate solution, immediately neutralized by 2 M Tris base, and finally lyophilized. Total IgG were purified with protein A-Sepharose following standard procedures [9]. After elution from beads, IgG fractions were dialyzed against PBS, sterile filtered, and $CaCl_2$ was added to a final concentration of 0.5 mM.

In Vitro Model of PV Using Keratinocyte Monolayers

HaCaT cells, a human immortalized keratinocyte cell line capable of forming normally differentiated epidermis [102], or primary keratinocytes isolated from oral mucosa, were used as an *in vitro* model of skin. HaCaT cells were grown as monolayer in Dulbecco's modified Eagle's medium (DMEM) supplemented with 10% FBS, penicillin (50 U/ml), streptomycin (50 µg/ml) and fungizone (2.5 µg/ml) in a humidified atmosphere with 5% CO_2. In some experiments, cells were cultured in serum-free keratinocyte growth medium (KGM) supplemented with growth factors plus antibiotics/antimycotic. Primary human keratinocytes were isolated from tongue specimens of patients undergoing glossoplasty. Each specimen was rinsed in phosphate-buffered saline (PBS) and submerged for 30 min in Dulbecco's modified Eagle's medium (DMEM) with 3% antibiotics/antimycotic. Epithelial sheet was partially separated from the connective tissues after 2h incubation in dispase at 4°C. Keratinocytes were isolated by treatment in 0.25% trypsin for 30 min at 37°C and plated in modified FAD (F12 and DMEM) medium supplemented with 20% fetal bovine serum (FBS), penicillin (50 U/ml), streptomycin (50 µg/ml) and fungizone (2.5 µg/ml). FAD was than changed with serum-free KGM. For reproducing the *in vitro* model of PV on cellcultures, keratinocytes were plated in 6-well dishes and incubated with 30% (v/v), 50% (v/v) sera in serum-free DMEM, whole unconcentrated sera, or threefold concentrated sera, depending on the experimental point being addressed.

In Vitro Models with Mouse Skin Organ Cultures

Mouse skin for organ cultures was taken from abdomen of 12-hour-old pups by punch biopsy. Each specimen was rinsed in phosphate-buffered saline

(PBS) and submerged for 30 min in Dulbecco's modified Eagle's medium (DMEM) with 10% antibiotics/antimycotic (Gibco BRL, Gaithersburg, MD). Then, specimens were directly subjected to experimental procedures by exposing them to 3-fold concentrated or unconcentrated 50% (v/v) whole sera in modified FAD (*F*12 *a*nd *D*MEM) medium [103].

In Vivo Passive Transfer of Sera Using Neonatal Mice

This study was conducted according to the Guidelines for Animal Experiments of the American Heart Association and rules of the National Institutes of Health (NIH publication No. 85-23, revised 1985) and approved by the scientific committee of the Regional Center on Craniofacial Malformations. All efforts were made to minimize the number of animals used and their suffering. Eight to twelve-hour-old neonatal balb/c mice were injected intraperitoneally or subcutaneously through a 30-gauge needle with 150µl tenfold concentrated sera. After 12 hours, the animals were subjected to gentle scraping of the lumbar skin to induce eventually the Nikolskiy phenomenon, then, 24 hours after injection, mice were evaluated for macroscopic blistering. Biopsies were taken by perilesional areas, if any, by using a standard 5 mm skin biopsy punch. After rinsing in PBS, these skin samples were immediately fixed in 10% formalin for regular histological analysis.

Standard Immunofluorescence Microscopy and Histology

Conventional immunofluorescence studies were carried out according to standard procedures. Cells were grown on glass coverslips and incubated in the presence of PV or normal sera as detailed above. Cells fixed in cold 100% methanol for 5 min or 4% paraformaldehyde for 10 min were then subjected to immunofluorescence. After washing with PBS, cells were permeabilized with 0,1% Triton X-100 for 5 min on ice and then washed three times in PBS containing 2% BSA to block non-specific sites. Samples were incubated with the appropriate primary antibody (i.e. anti-pancytokeratin, or anti-Dsg3 diluted 1:10 in 3% BSA/PBS) for 1h on ice, and washed in BSA/PBS twice. Finally, cells were exposed to specie-specific antibodies (1:100) conjugated to FITC or Texas Red (Dako Denmark A/S). In some experiments, cells were directly incubated with anti-human IgG to investigate deposits of of serum antibodies in the intercellular space. Nuclei were stained with Hoechst 33342 (5 μg/ml) on formaldehyde-fixed cells. Note that all steps were performed keeping keratinocytes on ice to block cellular metabolism. Specimens were examined with a Zeiss Axiophot microscope (Calr Zeiss Inc., Thornwood, NY) at x 400 magnification and fluorescence images were acquired with an Evolution VF fast digital camera (MediaCybernetics, UK).

For histological analysis, tissue samples were fixed in 10% formalin, processed for paraffine sectioning, and stained with hematoxylin and eosin by routine methods [104].

Evaluatiotion of Acantholysis in Cell Monolayers

Morphology
Specific changes in cytoskeleton organization, such as retraction of keratin filaments from cell borders onto nucleus, and detachment of keratinocytes from one another evaluated by staining of desmosomal components such as Dsg3, both have been considered as the hallmarks of pemphigus acantholysis *in vitro*.

Morphometric Analysis
The extent of cell detachment (acantholysis) in cell monolayers was measured by modifying previously published protocols [91]. Cells were subjected to immunofluorescence procedures and the images of ten representative microscopic fields were recorded. The percentage of acantholysis in each field observed by immunofluorescence was computed (Adobe Photoshop) by subtracting the percentage of the area covered by the cells from the total areas of the microscopic field, taken as 100%.

Results

Selection of Patients and Characterization of Sera

PV patients enrolled for the study were not taking corticosteroids at the time of serum collection. On clinical examination, they showed painful buccal erosions (n=4) and two of them also exhibited skin involvement. In the patient reported in figure 1, oral lesions involved gums, cheek, tongue, and lips (Figure 1. (a)). He presented crusted papules on the extensor surfaces of the forearms, chest, and upper back (Figure 1. (c,d,e)); also the genital region was interested by erosive lesions (Figure 1. (b)).

Indirect immunofluorescence (IIF) on monkey oesophagus - showing intercellular deposits of IgG, and histology – displaying a suprabasal intra-epithelial cleft, confirmed the diagnosis of PV (Figure 2. (a,b)). Immunoreactivity of sera on our cell culture system was then tested by immunofluorescence on HaCaT monolayers and confirmed by Western blot analysis. PV IgG, but not IgG of control sera, described the typical fishnet-like pattern all around the surface of keratinocytes, indicating that PV IgG targeted antigen(s) located in the intercellular substance (ICS) (Figure 2. (c,d)). Immunoprecipitation of HaCaT extracts with PV sera followed by Western blotting of the resulting immunocomplexes revealed that IgG from PV sera recognized Dsg3 (n=4, 100%) and Dsg1 (n=2, 50%) (Figure 2. (e,f)). Consistent with the known correspondence between clinical phenotype and autoantibody profile, serum IgG from patients with mucosal PV bound desmoglein 3, whereas those from PV patients having cutaneous involvement reacted with Dsg1 in addition to Dsg3 (Figure 2. (e)).

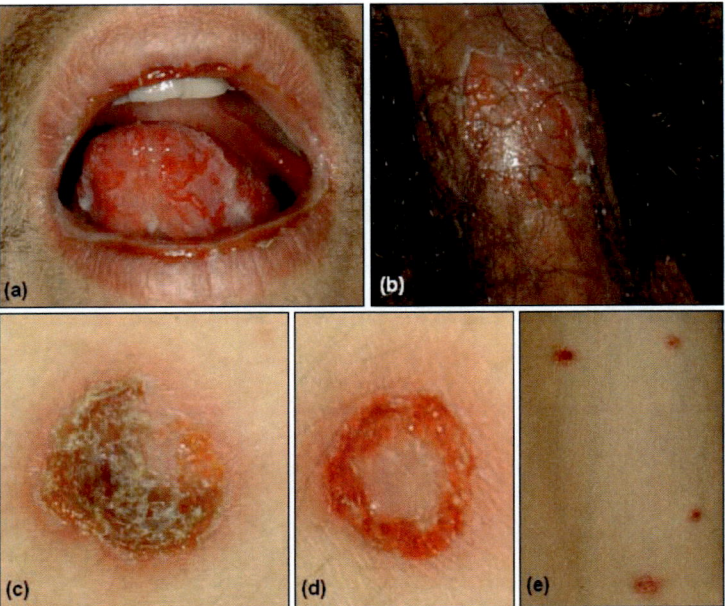

Figure 1. Oral (a) and genital (b) involvement of the lesions. The patient presented crusted papules and on the skin of the upper back (c), extensor surfaces of the forearms (d), and chest (e).

Thus, for our experiments, we used sera from two patients with PV mucosal dominant type (PV2, PV3), two with the mucocutaneous type of PV (PV1, PV4), and three healthy donors. All PV sera tested were found to describe similar immunostaining on keratinocytes irrespective of whether they were taken from patients with mucosal dominant rather than mucocutaneous types of PV (not shown). Furthermore, the catalogue of potential self antigens immunoprecipitated by PV IgG included a number of molecules with different relative molecular masses (Figure 2. (g)).

PV Serum Induces Specific Changes in KIF Arrangement

We first reproduced what is considered the classic *in vitro* model of PV. In HaCaT cells, KIF-labelling FITC fluorescence was predominant along cell periphery, as diffuse green spots on the entire cortical cytoplasm (Figure 3. (a)). Keratinocytes were treated with 50% normal or PV sera for 48h, a time period wherein morphologic changes become usually visible [105].

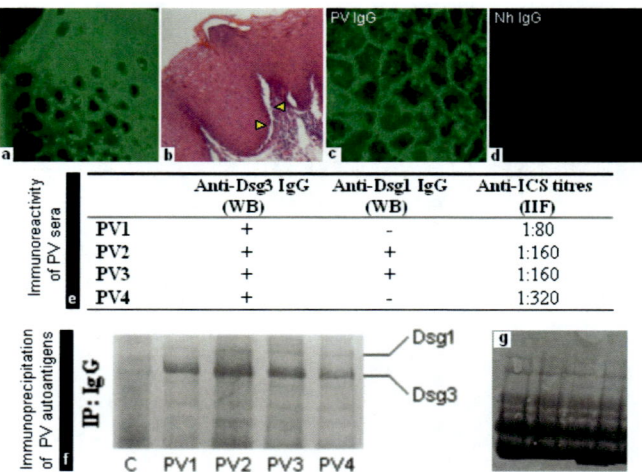

Figure 2. Immunoreactivity of sera. Histological examination of oral perilesional tissues from patient PV1 shows suprabasilar acantholysis (b). The presence of anti-intercellular substance (ICS) IgG in PV sera was probed by immunofluorescence on monkey oesophagus (a,e). Immunoreactivity of sera against HaCaT proteins revealed that PV IgG (c), but not normal human (Nh) IgG (d), immunostained antigen(s) located in the ICS of HaCaT keratinocytes. Reactivity of PV IgG against Dsg1 and Dsg3 from HaCaT cell lysates was assessed by Western blotting (e,f). SDS-PAGE of the immunocomplexes stained with Ponceau red (g).

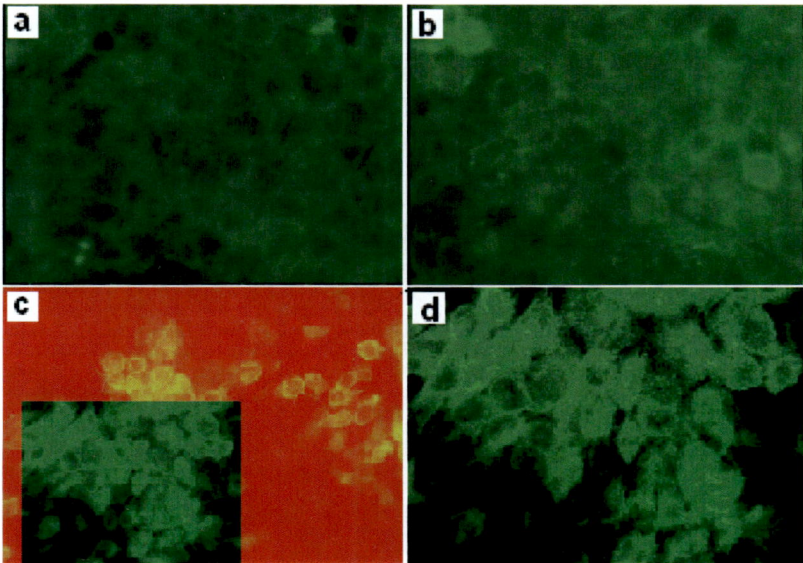

Figure 3. Cytokeratin staining of HaCaT cells cultured for 48 hours in normal conditions (a) or exposed to normal (b) or PV sera (c), reveals that PV serum induce specific changes of keratin cytoskeleton. As shown in the higher magnification photograph (d), the cells round up, keratins detach from membrane and collapse onto the nuclei.

Indeed, keratinocytes exposed to PV serum (n=4) displayed KIF retraction and rounding up (Figure 3. (c,d)), whereas untreated cells (n=3) or those incubated with normal sera (n=3) did not exhibit changes in cytokeratin staining (Figure 3. (b)). Our data suggest that PV sera can specifically induce keratin cytoskeleton reorganization and cell-cell detachment.

Detection of Acantholysis Induced by Concentrated PV Sera through Dsg3 Staining

HaCaT monolayers were exposed to threefold concentrated or unconcentrated PV and control sera for 24, 48, and 72 hours, then we tested the ability of whole PV sera to induce acantholysis in our experimental conditions. Immunofluorescence performed on cultured HaCaT revealed that incubation with 30% concentrated PV serum within 24 h induced retraction of keratin filaments (KIF) from cell borders (Figure 4. (a,b)) which is considered the hallmark of pemphigus acantholysis [40].

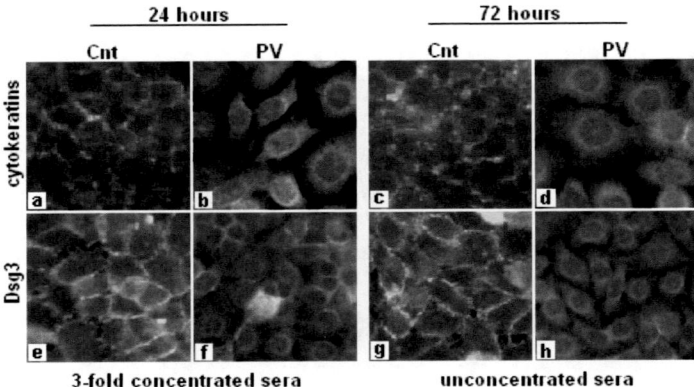

Figure 4. As revealed by immunofluorescence microscopy, threefold concentrated PV sera, but not control sera, induced KIFs retraction (*a,b*) and disruption of cell-cell contacts (*e,f*) within 24 h. The same morphological changes were observed by using unconcentrated sera (*c,d,g,h*), although keratinocyte acantholytic dysmorphisms became evident 72 h after treatment.

Unconcentrated PV sera induced KIF retraction as well, but the earliest events were seen after 48 h (not shown) and become clear 72 h after exposure to PV sera (Figure 4. (c,d)). Cell-cell contacts were also studied by immunostaining Dsg3 with the 5H10 monoclonal antibody. Dsg3 was seen redistributed on cell surface with a dynamic similar to that observed for KIF (Figure 4. (e-h)). Taken together, these data demonstrate that whole PV serum can induce specific acantholytic changes on keratinocytes *in vitro*, such as KIF retraction and Dsg3 redistribution. Furthermore, we conclude that Dsg3 staining may be used for detection of acantholytic cells *in vitro*.

In Vitro Model of PV with Mouse Skin Cultures

To assess the ability of PV sera to induce the histological changes of acantholysis, e.g. detachment of suprabasal keratinocytes from the basal-cell line, we established organotypic cultures from mouse skin and then incubated them with 50% (v/v) PV or normal sera for 24 and 48 hours. Histological analysis revealed that, within 48 h, all PV sera (n=4), but no control sera (n=3), were able to induce intraepithelial detachment occurring just above the basal-cell layer, a typical finding of PV acantholysis (Figure 5. (a,b)). Thus, we concluded that the use of whole PV serum can model the disease *in vitro* in skin organ cultures.

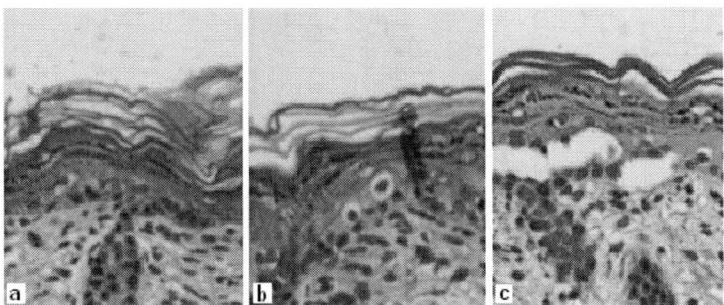

Figure 5. Organ cultures were established from skin tissues of neonatal mice (a) and then exposed to PV (c) or normal (b) sera. Histological analysis on skin organ cultures show the intraepithelial cleft typical of pemphigus in samples incubated with PV (c) but not normal (b) sera.

In Vivo Model of PV with Passive Transfer of Sera in Neonatal Mice

We established an *in vivo* model of PV as follows. Eight to twelve-hour-old balb/c mice were injected subcutaneously with 150 µl 10-fold concentrated PV or control sera. Mice receiving PV sera (n=4), but not controls (n=3), showed pemphigus-like skin blisters on about 24 hours after injection (Figure 6. (a,b)). At this time, skin samples were excised by standard punch biopsy and epithelial sheets were fixed and processed for histology as detailed in materials and methods. Histological analysis showed lower acantholysis, a common finding of PV lesions (Figure 6. (c,d)). Taken together, these data showed that mice receiving whole PV serum can reproduce both clinical and histological features of PV.

Discussion

In the present chapter we assessed the pathogenicity of whole PV sera taken from patients in the active phase of disease in both *in vitro* and *in vivo* models. Consistent with the idea that serum factors other than IgG can play a role in PV pathogenesis, we therefore sought to test whether whole PV sera were able to reproduce the clinical, histological and cytological changes of the disease, in order to propose these models for future studies on PV. Results clearly showed that, in our experimental conditions, whole PV serum is able to induce acantholysis both *in vitro* and *in vivo*.

Across the last decades, PV autoantibodies have been shown to be pathogenic in that they induced blister formation in skin organ cultures [106] and neonatal mice [98]. Also, purified PV IgG have been usually utilized for inducing acantholytic changes in keratinocyte monolayers [88]. In recent years, monoclonal antibodies against either Dsg3 or Dsg1 have been proposed, which should reproduce the pathophysiology of pemphigus within experimental models [99, 103]. However, the lack of spontaneous blistering in the mouse model injected with anti-Dsg3 antibody alone as well as the finding that mice immunized with full-length Dsg3 did not develop lesions [107] suggest caution. With regard to this, it should be taken into account that epitope specificity of the antibodies could be critical in inducing blister formation. Indeed, it seems that pathogenic PV IgG recognize linear and conformational epitopes formed by the N-terminal 161 amino acids of Dsg3 containing sequences functionally crucial for cadherin-mediated cell-cell adhesion [18].

In addition, autoimmunity in pemphigus seems to be not just restricted to desmogleins. Besides the sporadic presence in PV patients of IgG against plakoglobin [21], desmoplakin [23], and desmocollins [22], indeed, compelling evidence now attests to the role of IgG against keratinocyte cholinergic receptors in the pathogenesis of acantholysis [25, 27].

Hence, a first approach to our reasoning should suggest the use of PV IgG, but not Dsg3-specific autoantibodies, in preparing the experimental model of PV. But are the concentration of IgG routinely used actually appropriate to mimic the disease? The amount of purified PV IgG usually chosen for *in vivo* experiments is very high, corresponding to a concentration 10-20-fold greater than that of physiologically occurring serum gamma globulins. In fact, neonatal mice are generally injected with 10-fold concentrated immune sera or 10 mg PV IgG per g of body weight - in comparison with 0.5-1mg /g normally occurring in humans [108]. It is emblematic that in neonatal mice receiving lower concentrations of PV IgG (2.5 mg/g) blister formation is delayed and complement appears to participate to the pathophysiology of acantholysis, whereas pups injected with 5-15 mg/g PV IgG rapidly develop extensive blisters without involvement, it seems, of any serum factor [109]. Clearly, the levels of human versus mouse PV IgG are not well comparable, as the skin bioavailability of IgG from either intraperitoneally or subcutaneously injected mice differs from that observed when IgG stem from plasma. However, anti-ICS IgG are easily revealed in mouse skin injected with unconcentrated whole

PV sera (Cirillo et al., unpublished), suggesting that physiologically occurring concentrations of PV IgG are able to bind epidermal antigen(s) within the target organ. Accordingly, one can speculate that blisters form in experimental PV because of the dramatic impact of exceedingly high doses of PV IgG on keratinocytes. The evidence of the subsequent blister formation could obscure the importance of factors other than IgG in PV pathogenesis, yet, these factors could participate as "supporting actors" in inducing blistering of PV patients' epidermis. In fact, pemphigus acantholysis is related to a series of cytokines, as detailed in the Introduction. Although these molecules are unlikely to be pathogenic by theirselves, they could be critical in regulating the delicate equilibrium ensuring the maintenance of cell adhesion. Furthermore, serum could be essential for the activation of Dsg3-targetting proteases such as matrix metalloproteinase (MMP) 9, whose role in PV acantholysis has been recently suggested [110]. Keratinocyte apoptosis too, which occurs both in PV patients' epidermis and PV sera-treated cell monolayers, seems to require serum factors other than IgG. Indeed, findings of two independent groups indicate that FasL, whose levels are significantly high in sera of untreated PV patients, plays a critical, maybe pathogenic role in the mechanisms underlying acantholysis [35, 111, 112]. Hence, the second point arising from our reasoning is whether using whole sera in place of PV IgG can be a better way to model the disease.

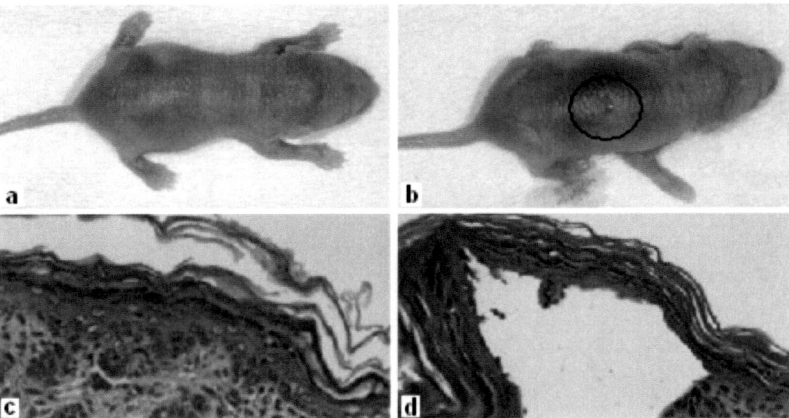

Figure 6. Clinical and histological features in the neonatal mouse model of pemphigus. Mice injected with PV sera developed pemphi-gus like-lesions on clinical esamination (*b*). Microscopically, peri-lesional skin showed low acantholysis (*d*). None of the above lesions were observed in mice receiving normal sera (*a,c*).

In vitro, we established PV models by using both human keratinocyte monolayers and mouse skin organ cultures. We did not utilized organotypic cultures from human tissues because the pathogenicity of whole PV serum on this tissue system has been assessed previously [100]. In cultured keratinocytes, the retraction of KIF onto nucleus is considered as a distinctive sign - the hallmark - of pemphigus acantholysis [67]. In skin organ cultures, the histological picture overlaps that observed *in vivo*, being represented by intraepithelial cleft within the parabasal layers of the epidermis. In both experimental systems, whole PV serum has been shown to reproduce the typical features of PV.

For the *in vivo* study, we utilized the neonatal mouse model by passive transfer of whole sera in place of purified PV IgG or anti-Dsg3 antibodies. Balb/c pups were injected with 10-fold concentrated PV serum. Once more, our experimental approach demonstrated that whole PV serum can induce pemphigus-like lesions *in vivo*.

As mentioned above, the use of PV serum to experimentally reproduce the disease stems from the idea that, besides the pivotal role of PV IgG, other serum factors such as cytokines can take a part in the pathogenesis of PV acantholysis. In other words, cytokines may act as "precipitating factors" leading the delicate equilibrium of cell-cell adhesion towards blister formation rather than maintenance of epithelial integrity, although further studies are needed to address this hypothesis. However, our investigation is important in that it enables researchers to use whole sera for studying the pathophysiology of PV, without leaving serum factors other than IgG out of consideration.

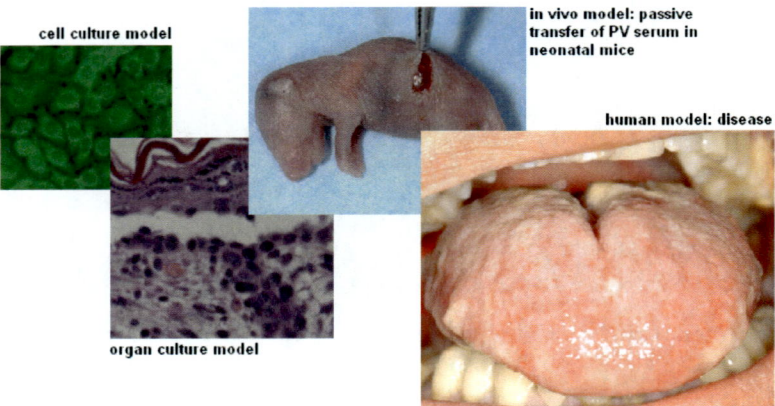

Figure7. Models of pemphigus.

On the basis of the above observations and those from our laboratories (Figure 7), we believe that the use of whole sera from patients with active PV - the only ones ensuring actual pathogenicity due to their ability to cause blister formation in humans - represents the most faithful manner to experimentally reproduce the disease. On these premises, in the present chapter we attempted to establish *in vitro* – both on keratinocyte monolayers and skin organ cultures – and *in vivo* models of pemphigus vulgaris by using whole PV sera from patients with active disease.

Chapter 3

Optimization of the Experimental Procedures: Semi-Quantitative LCIF Microscopy, Cirillo's HSU Buffer, KAD Medium

The hallmark of PV acantholysis *in vitro* is considered the retraction of keratin intermediate filaments (KIF) onto the nucleus, which parallels with loss of cell-cell adhesion and rounding up of keratinocytes.

However, the fine morphological changes of keratinocytes as well as the fate of cell adhesion structures cannot be appreciated on immunofluorescence by the simple cytokeratin staining.

Here we show that acantholytic dysmorphisms are sharply investigated by using PV IgG as a primary antibody on metabolically quiescent living cells. Indeed, PV IgG recognize a wide spectrum of molecules and enabled us to monitor the main changes occurring in acantholytic keratinocytes, including cell shrinkage with the appearance of prickle-like processes, detachment of keratinocytes from one another, and collapse of cytoskeleton-bound proteins along nuclear periphery. This method has wider applications as it could be useful for staining cell periphery of keratinocytes and changes in cell shape.

Furthermore, images displayed clear and sharp contours, because living cell microscopy allows to avoid antigen distortion due to cell manipulation which usually precedes the immunolabeling.

Introduction

In pemphigus, intraepithelial cleft develops as a consequence of the loss of cell-cell adhesion among keratinocytes, or acantholysis [1]. When acantholytic, the epithelial cells become rounded, with the cytoplasm contracted round the nucleus, and often form small groups within a vesicle. Immunofluorescence studies have revealed that PV serum autoantibodies bind antigens located within the intercellular substance of keratinocytes [3] and they usually correlate with the extent and the activity of the disease [7].

Dsg1/3 extracellular domains are critically involved in maintaining intercellular contacts mediated by desmosomes [14]. By anchoring the intermediate filament cytoskeleton to sites of cell-cell adhesion, desmosomes form a highly resilient, supracellular network which is required for tissue integrity. Although the binding of Dsg3 to keratin intermediate filaments (KIF) is mediated by a number of structural and adapter proteins that work intracellularly (including plakoglobin and the plakin family proteins, e.g. desmoplakin I/II, plakophilins, envoplakin and periplakin), the stability of desmosome is largely dependent by the structural and functional integrity of the desmoglein extracellular domain [40].

As this intercellular fraction of Dsg3 hold the main epitopes recognized by PV IgG, acantholysis could be due to the simple perturbation of Dsg3 adhesion function through steric hindrance [2]. After pemphigus IgG binding to their desmosomal targets, cell surface Dsg1/3 – prevalently the unassembled clusters – are thought to be partially internalized [113]. Finally, loss of cell-cell adhesion in PV is likely to take place when keratinocytes become unable in maintaining steady-state levels of Dsg3 [105]. Alternatively, proteinases such as matrix metalloproteinase (MMP)-9 may specifically digest Dsg3 extracellular domain [94, 110]. In any case, when Dsg3 function is impaired, keratin filament are thought to collapse onto nucleus and determine keratinocytes to round up. Indeed, KIF retraction is considered the hallmark of PV acantholysis *in vitro* [67].

However, as emerged from our personal experience, staining of cytokeratins on formalin-fixed cells has revealed unexpected difficulties and sometimes disappointing results. To eliminate experienced shortcomings in documenting the effect of PV serum by IF microscopy, here we propose a novel and useful method to stain acantholytic cells on keratinocyte monolayers. As a prerequisite to address the above questions, we have evaluated the expression levels of Dsg1 under different culture conditions, in order to prepare cells endogenously enriched in Dsg1.

Materials and Methods

Culture Conditions and *In Vitro* Models

HaCaT cells were cultured as reported in chapter 2. Cells from T-75 flasks were plated on 35 mm Petri dishes and grown to semi-confluence in complete DMEM in an atmosphere humidified with 5% CO_2. To assess the expression of Dsg1 under different culture conditions, cells were seeded and grown to confluence for 7 days in 6-well dishes by using different media, namely: DMEM, Ham F12, FAD (F12+DMEM), McCoy's, RPMI, keratinocyte growth medium (KGM), KAD (KGM+DMEM).

KAD medium, consisting of a mixture (1:1) of keratinocyte growth medium (KGM) supplemented with growth factors and DMEM plus 10% FBS, was supplemented with penicillin (50 U/ml), streptomycin (50 µg/ml) and fungizone (2.5 µg/ml). When treating cells with human sera, FBS-free KAD was used [103].

Western Blot Analysis and Immunoprecipitation

Adherent cells were rinsed with complete PBS and scraped in PBS containing the protease inhibitor phenylmethylsulfonylfluoride (PMSF) at 1 mM. Pellets obtained after centrifugation at 4°C at 800 x g for 10 minutes were suspended in Triton buffer (20mM Tris-HCl, pH 7.5, 150 mM NaCl, 5 mM EDTA, 1% Triton X-100, 1 mM DTT, 1 mM PMSF, 10 µg/ml leupeptin and 10 µg/ml aprotinin) and centrifuged for 30 min at 16,000 g: the supernatant was transferred to a fresh tube and stored as triton soluble pool. Pellets were then solubilized in SDS buffer (20mM Tris-HCl, pH 7.5, 150 mM NaCl, 5 mM EDTA, 0.5% SDS, 1% Triton X-100, 1 mM DTT, 1 mM PMSF, 10 µg/ml leupeptin and 10 µg/ml aprotinin). Alternatively, triton-insoluble pellets were resuspended in high salt-urea (HSU) buffer (50 mM HEPES, 800 mM NaCl, 6 M urea, 0.2% Triton X-100, 1 mM DTT, 1 mM PMSF, 10 µg/ml leupeptin and 10 µg/ml aprotinin) and stored as C-HSU soluble cell lysates.

Proteins subjected to immunoprecipitation were extracted by using the IP buffer (50mM Tris-HCl, pH 7.5, 150 mM NaCl, 0.5% Nonidet P-40, 1 mM DTT, 1 mM PMSF) and separated by 8% sodium dodecyl sulphate (SDS)-polyacrylamide gel electrophoresis (PAGE). The immunoreactivity of PV IgG against Dsg1 and Dsg3 was essayed by combined immunoprecipitation-western blotting, following the procedures reported by Cirillo and colleagues [105, 114].

In Vitro Model of PV Using Cultured Keratinocytes

We have exposed cultured cells to PV patients' sera as proposed originally by Swanson and Dahl on skin organ cultures [100], adapting the standard protocols to keratinocyte monolayers (see chapter 2).

For reproducing the *in vitro* model of PV on cells cultures, keratinocytes were incubated with either threefold concentrated or unconcentrated 30% (v/v) sera from PV patients and controls for different time periods, as specified in the results section.

Specific changes in cytoskeleton organization, such as retraction of keratin filaments from cell borders onto nucleus, and detachment of keratinocytes from one another evaluated by staining of desmosomal components recognized by PV IgG, both have been investigated and compared.

Semiquantitative Living Cell Immunofluorescence (LCIF) Microscopy

We have previously published the procedures for LCIF [115] and for semiquantitative analysis [116]. Cells were grown on glass coverslips and incubated in the presence or absence of normal or PV sera.

After washing with PBS, cells were permeabilized with 0,1% Triton X-100 for 5 min on ice and then washed three times in PBS containing 2% BSA to block non-specific sites. Samples were incubated with the appropriate primary antibody (i.e. anti-pancytokeratin, anti-Dsg3 or PV IgG diluted 1:10 in 3% BSA/PBS) for 1h on ice, washed in BSA/PBS, and fixed in cold 100% methanol for 5 min or 4% paraformaldehyde for 10 min. Finally, cells were exposed to specie-specific antibodies (1:100) conjugated to FITC (Dako Denmark A/S).

In some experiments, cells were directly incubated with anti-human IgG to investigate deposits of PV autoantibodies. Nuclei were stained with Hoechst 33342 (5 µg/ml) on formaldehyde-fixed cells. Note that all steps were performed keeping keratinocytes on ice to block cellular metabolism.

Specimens were examined with a Zeiss Axiophot microscope (Calr Zeiss Inc., Thornwood, NY) at 400X magnification and fluorescence images were acquired with an Evolution VF fast digital camera (MediaCybernetics, Wokingham Berkshire, UK).

Note that samples were processed simultaneously and photographic procedures held constant to obtain semiquantitative results.

Results

Optimization of Extraction Rate and Expression Levels of Dsgs

We first compared the ability of SDS-buffer and C-HSU-buffer in extracting triton-insoluble Dsg3 from cell lysates. Apoptosis was induced in keratinocytes through staurosporine (REF) and differential protein extraction was carried out. After discarding the triton-soluble pools, the resulting pellets were solubilized either in SDS buffer or in C-HSU buffer, separated with SDS-PAGE, and then subjected to Western blotting. Results demonstrated C-HSU buffer to be highly effective in extracting triton-insoluble Dsg3 (Figure 1). The appearance of apoptotic fragments was detectable with both buffers, although the signals was stronger by using SDS-buffer. The quality of bands resulted, however, very weak (Figure 1(a)).

Then, to obtain robust levels of endogenously-expressed Dsg1, we cultured HaCaT for 7 days with different media and than expression of desmogleins was evaluated by Western blot analysis. Cells cultured in KAD showed higher levels of Dsg1 than those grown in DMEM (Figure 2.(a), lanes 1 and 7) while the other tested media seemed to be not effective in promoting the endogenous synthesis of Dsg1.

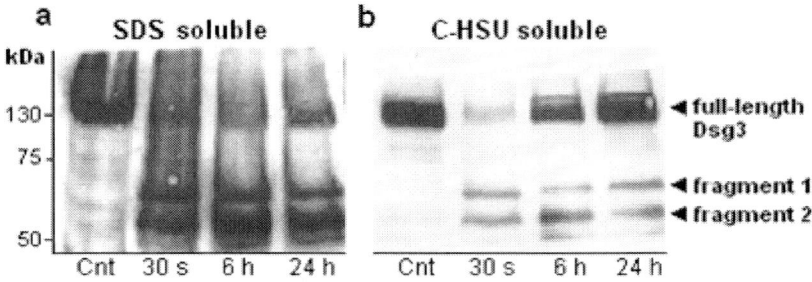

Figure 1. Western blotting on triton-insoluble pool of protein as SDS soluble (a) or C-HSU soluble (b) fractions. Cell lysates were established from keratino-cytes undergoing STS-induced apoptosis.

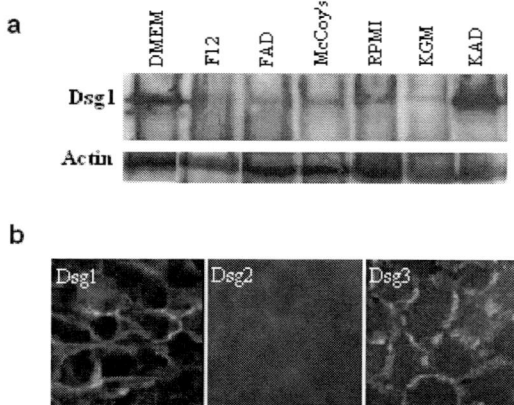

Figure 2. (a) Dsg1 levels assessed by western blot analysis. KAD medium was effective in increasing the amount of Dsg1 in cultured cells, if compared with standard media. (b) As revealed by immunofluorescence, cells cultured 7 days with KAD expressed high levels of Dsg1 and Dsg3, whereas Dsg2 was virtually undetectable. In this stage of differentiation, desmoglein pattern was similar to that observed in the stratum granulosum of the epidermis, the site of blister formation in PF. Figures are representative of three independent experiments.

At the selected stage of differentiation, KAD-cultured HaCaT expressed well detectable levels of Dsg1 and Dsg3, whereas Dsg2 was virtually absent (Figure 2.b). Indeed, KAD medium was effective in promoting sustained expression of Dsg3 in addition to Dsg1 (not shown). Thus, we carried out most experiments by culturing cells with KAD to induce sustained expression of Dsgs.

Cell-Cell Detachment and KIF Collapse Can Be Revealed by PV Igg Staining

In chapter 2, we have reproduced what is considered the classic *in vitro* model of PV. In HaCaT cells, KIF labelling FITC-fluorescence was predominant along cell periphery, as diffuse green spots on the entire cortical cytoplasm. However, cytokeratin labelling was slightly blurred in the majority of control samples as well as in some PV treated cells (n=2, not shown). Furthermore, as in keratinocytes exposed to PV serum the intracellular network formed by keratins collapsed onto nucleus, cellular borders and/or residual contacts among acantholytic cells appeared hardly detectable (Figures

3, 4 *chapter 2*). Thus, although keratin staining is effective in highlighting acantholytic changes, however, photograms are not always of reproducible quality and do not allow for labeling intercellular contact areas. To investigate the effects of PV serum on cell morphology by using PV IgG as a primary antibody, we determined optimal conditions in pilot assays and then we carried out extensive experiments by diluting PV IgG 1:10, as reported in materials and methods. Keratinocytes were treated with 30% (v/v) PV or normal sera for 72h and then morphology was investigated through living cell immunofluorescence microscopy. Dramatic changes in cell shape were observed in keratinocytes exposed to PV but not normal sera (Figure 3).

These dysmorphisms paralleled with profound redistribution of PV IgG, which appeared to be markedly internalized. Nevertheless, cell borders were still clearly distinguishable. Interestingly, IgG staining also localized onto nuclear periphery as a slight green fluorescence of oval shape (Figure 3, arrows), resembling KIF arrangement during acantholysis. This finding may be explained by the fact that Dsg3 undergoing internalization remains partially bound to keratin cytoskeleton.

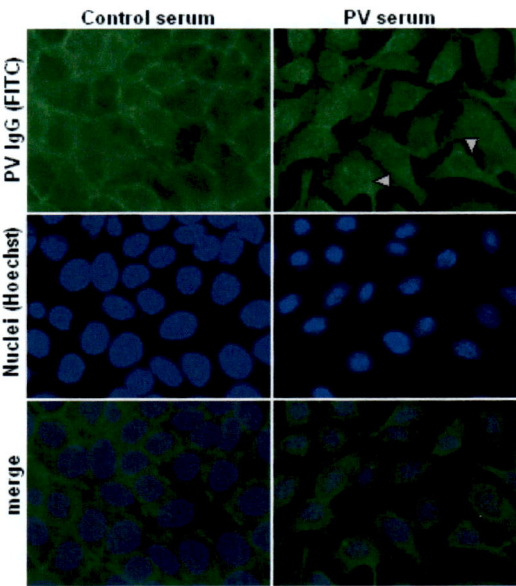

Figure 3. Cell-cell detachment occurring after a 72-hour exposition to PV, but not control sera. As shown by immunofluorescence microscopy, the use of PV IgG as a primary antibody on living but metabolically quiescent cells allow an optimal resolution of cell contours, adhesion areas, and nuclear periphery.

Thus, staining of acantholytic keratinocytes with PV IgG by living cell immunofluorescence microscopy appeared to fulfil all the well-established hallmarks of pemphigus, that is cell-cell detachment, rounding up, and collapse of cytoskeleton-associated proteins onto nucleus.

Time-Course of PV-Induced Acantholytic Dysmorphisms on Keratinocytes

To study the morphological changes of keratinocytes accompanying the progressive loss of cell-cell adhesion, we used 3-fold concentrated 30% PV sera, which are known to induce acantholysis within 24 h (Cirillo et al., unpublished).

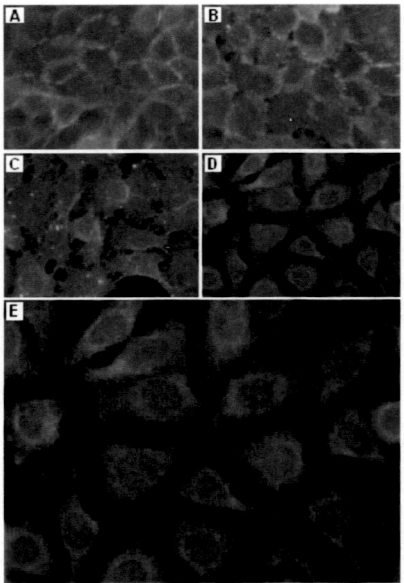

Figure 4. Phenomenology of cell-cell detachment as revealed by living cell immunofluorescence microscopy. To emphasize the phenomena accompanying keratinocyte adhesion loss, cells were treated with 3-fold concentrated PV sera for 24 hours. First changes in cell shape became evident within 6 hours after treatment (B). Cell shrinkage and formation of prickle-like processes appeared within 12 hours (C), whereas 24 hours after incubation with PV serum cells were clearly detached from one another (D). At higher magnification, typical morphological changes of acantholytic cells were detectable (E), see text for details. Figures were representative of at least two independent experiments conducted by probing all sera.

Cell morphology was assessed through LCIM by using PV IgG as a primary antibody. Signs of cell shrinkage were appreciable within 6 h after treatment (Figure 4). Punctuate clusters of FITC-fluorescence on cell surface, referred to as contact areas among keratinocytes, appeared as elongated processes which brought together shrinking cells (Figure 4(b)). Cell dysmorphisms became obvious 12 h after treatment, and cell-cell adhesion structures immunostained by PV IgG assumed a prickle-like appearance (Figure 4(c)). After 24 h, keratinocytes were completely detached from one another (Figure 4(d)). Some cellular pocessess extending from keratinocyte surface were still recognizable; however, no signs of punctuate clusters were detectable. Furthermore, perinuclear localization of PV IgG was revealed as a sharp FITC fluorescence along nuclear periphery (Figure 4(e)), resembling those induced by keratin cytoskeleton collapse in acantholytic cells. Time-course experiments were also performed with control sera, but no morphological changes were revealed on immunofluorescence (not shown). Overall, these morphological analyses showed that immunolabelling with PV IgG represents an excellent method to follow acantholytic changes on keratinocytes.

Discussion

In the present chapter, we have shown that immunostaining of acantholytic keratinocytes with PV IgG is effective in following the cell fate in response to PV serum. Cell shrinkage, appearance of prickle-like processes and subsequent disruption of cell-cell contact areas, detachment of keratinocytes from one another, and collapse of cytoskeleton-bound proteins along nuclear periphery, all these acantholysis-associated phenomena were well detectable by living cell immunofluorescence microscopy using PV IgG as a primary antibody. We have also shown that C-HSU baffer is reliable for an effective solubilization of the triton-insoluble pool of Dsg3. Finally, KAD medium has been demonstrated to be useful in establishing Dsg-rich keratinocytes.

Although the main alteration of keratinocytes subjected to PV autoimmunity *in vitro* was represented by cell-cell detachment and rounding up, retraction of KIF from the cortical cytoplasm onto the nucleus has been considered as the hallmark of PV-induced acantholysis. However, cell contact areas as well as keratinocyte contours are not well investigable through cytokeratin labelling, principally because KIF loss their connections with the transmembrane adhesion proteins during acantholysis. On the contrary, deposits of PV IgG along cell surface as well as within the cytoplasm (resulting from PV IgG internalization together with PV antigens) made us able to stain both keratinocyte borders and residual cell-cell contact areas. Furthermore, as internalized desmogleins remain partially bound to keratin cytoskeleton during acantholysis, we were able to observe the collapse of presumptive KIF-associated desmogleins onto nucleus. We cannot predict whether these changes occur also *in vivo*, nor we actually know whether LCIM is applicable on fresh skin biopsy. However, the hallmark of PV acantholysis *in vivo* is well established, being represented by a gross phenomenon such as skin blistering, whose histological expression is epidermal splitting. Instead, the *in vitro* model of PV on cultured keratinocytes is still debated and it is reproduced in different manner according to each author's experience.

Under a methodological point of view, by incubating the primary antibody on living – although metabolically quiescent – cells, we reduced the potential distortion of the three-dimentional folding that cadherin are likely to undergo during fixation process. Despite living keratinocytes were incubated with non-ionic detergents to allow the penetration of PV IgG within the cell, no relevant alterations in morphology were seen in controls, suggesting that the permeabilization procedures in such quiescent cells do not remarkably affect their shape. However, when the staining of intracellular antigens is not required, permeabilization could be avoided to rule out the potential risk of causing alteration of cell shape. By and large, this method could be widely applied to detect keratinocyte shape and its changes. However, when studying PV acantholysis, the cells could be fixed and then directly incubated with the secondary antibody, as PV IgG are already bound to their antigen(s). It is worth of note that neither the anti-desmoglein antibody profile nor the anti-ICS titres did apparently affect the staining intensity, perhaps reflecting the saturation of binding sites for the FITC-conjugated secondary antibody due to the high serum concentration of PV IgG. Thus, neither a cut-off value of anti-ICS titres nor the precise immunoreactivity of such autoantibodies seems required to ensure a good staining of keratinocytes. This finding make LCIM an approachable research tool in order to ameliorate the study of PV pathophysiology and, more in general, the morphological changes in keratinocyte shape occurring in a lot of skin diseases or during biological phenomena such as apoptosis.

Keratinocyte outline and cell-cell contacts during acantholysis have been stained with antibodies against a number of cell adhesion proteins, including plakoglobin [67], desmoplakins [42], Dsg1 [117], Dsg3 [118], and E-cadherin

[89]. These proteins share a distribution usable for studying cell periphery and changes in cell shape because they are found prevalently within cell adhesion structures such as desmosomes and adherens junctions. IgG against PV antigens recognize mainly Dsg3 and Dsg1, although the spectrum of PV autoantigens is thought to encompass molecules other than desmogleins, such as acetylcholine receptors [25, 27]. Hence, immunostaining with PV IgG does not simply overlap that of Dsg3. Rather, it encompasses a number of proteins expressed on keratinocyte surface thus allowing a sharp and exact reproduction of cell periphery. For these reasons, we found it useful in all cases where following changes in cell shape is required.

In summary, here we showed as living cell immunofluorescence microscopy using PV IgG as a primary antibody can be useful to stain acantholytic dysmorphisms induced by PV sera on keratinocytes. In general, this method allows a sharp labelling of cell periphery and is recommended whenever keratinocyte shape and its changes need to be investigated.

Chapter 4

Study of Anti-Desmoglein Autoimmunity: Pemphigus Vulgaris as a Desmoglein-Remodeling Disease

Defects of cell-cell adhesion underlye disruption of epithelial integrity observed in patients with pemphigus vulgaris (PV). Pathogenic PV autoantibodies found in patients' sera target desmoglein 3 (Dsg3), but how does this phenomenon affect Dsg-dependent adhesion and participate to acantholysis still remains controversial. Here, we show that PV serum determines a reduction of Dsg3 half-life in HaCaT keratinocytes. We also reported that depletion of full-length Dsg3 could be due its progressive cleavage, leading to the formation of two fragmentation products with apparent molecular masses of about 60 kDa (fragment 1) and 70 kDa (fragment 2), as revealed by Western blotting. Immunofluorescence studies suggest that PV IgG exert their effect prevalently by binding non-desmosomal Dsg3 without causing its massive internalization. Furthermore, PV IgG targeting desmosome-assembled Dsg3 do not induce depletion of Dsg3 from the adhesion sites. Conversely, incorporation of PV IgG-Dsg3 complexes into new forming desmosomes appears perturbed. Similar behaviour was shown by Dsg1 when cells were subjected to anti-Dsg1 pemphigus autoimmunity. Next, we carried out more in-depth analysis on the Dsg3-depleting activity of PV sera, and focused on the role played by anti-Dsg3 IgG. The data demonstrate that anti-Dsg3 PV IgG recognizing non-conformational epitopes of Dsg3 are pathogenic solely when administered on doses largely exceeding those found in PV sera. Furthermore, our findings suggest that disruption of cell adhesion in PV is not the result of Dsg3 depletion, rather the latter may represent a late event in acantholysis.

Introduction

Desmoglein 3 (Dsg3) is the best characterized autoantigen of pemphigus vulgaris (PV) [10]. It is a 130-kDa desmosomal type I glycoprotein which is critically involved in ensuring calcium-dependent intercellular adhesion among keratinocytes [40]. Dsg3 is found in the basal and spinous layers of the epidermis and gradually diminishes as the cells became more differentiated, whereas in the oral mucosa Dsg3 is detected at high levels in all cell layers [20].

Indeed, mucosal PV associates with the presence of circulating IgG against linear and conformational epitopes of Dsg3 [16, 17]. Skin involvement and disease progression correlate with the appearance of IgG against Dsg1, a cell adhesion protein strictly related to Dsg3 [11]. Taken together, these observations led to the concept of desmoglein compensation as an explanation for acantholysis. Desmoglein compensation theory has also provided indirect support to the idea that PV IgG can cause direct inhibition of desmogleins' adhesive function through steric hindrance [2].

Alternatively, or additionally, binding of autoantibodies to Dsg3 could modulate its own synthesis, leading to the formation of aberrant desmosomes lacking Dsg3 both *in vitro* [42] and *in vivo* [43]. However, biochemical studies focused on Dsg3 turn-over in normal and pathologic conditions are still lacking.

To date, it is not yet clear whether PV IgG are able to bind desmosome-assembled Dsg3 or block its extracellular domain before Dsg3 engages contacts with apposed cells and, however, it remains to address whether these interactions can cause desmosome splitting or prevent formation of new desmosomes, respectively. With regard to this, it is worth of note that detachment of keratinocytes from each other seems to occur first in the interdesmosomal areas, while desmosomes appear to separate only in the late acantholysis [95]. It has been recently suggested that PV IgG may work through the depletion of Dsg3 from keratinocytes, possibly depriving cell from free Dsg3 before its assembly into desmosomes [119]. However, the final event leading to abrogation of Dsg3 from the cell in response to PV serum is still unknown.

Recent studies reported the presumptive depletion of Dsg3 from desmosomes to depend on the pathogenicity of mouse anti-Dsg3 IgG against conformational epitopes of Dsg3 [119]. This finding would be in agreement with previous papers demonstrating that the dominant autoimmune epitopes in PV are found in the N-terminal adhesive surfaces of Dsg3 [17].

By using domain-swapped Dsg3 recombinants, indeed, Futei and colleagues showed that the majority of autoimmune IgG in PV sera reacted with epitopes formed by aa 1-161 of the NH_2-terminus of Dsg3 [16]. IgG against the amino-terminal adhesive interface of Dsg3 were subsequently found to be pathogenic [18]. In general, the role of IgG against conformational sequences of the extracellular domain of Dsg3 in PV has received great attention.

In marked contrast, participation of Dsg3 linear epitopes in PV remains largely unknown. The recent finding that IgG titres against a small stretch of the NH_2-terminus of Dsg3 are associated with active PV [120], however, is relevant to this regard. Indeed, IgG in the PV sera detect non-conformational epitopes of Dsg3 in addition to the previously identified conformation-dependent ones. However, the pathophysiological significance of these above-mentioned anti-Dsg3 IgG is still obscure.

In the present chapter, we sought to determine whether autoantibodies from PV sera *(a)* induce alterations of Dsg3 turn-over, *(b)* deplete Dsg3 from assembled desmosomes or cause their splitting and/or *(c)* prevent the recruitment of PV IgG-bound Dsg3 into desmosomes. An additional endpoint was *(d)* to investigate the fate of Dsg3 during PV acantholysis. Parallel studies were also conducted on Dsg1 as a comparison.

Then, we focused on the action of Dsg3-targeting IgG in the attempt to investigate the presumptive pathogenicity of anti-Dsg3 antibodies purified from patients' sera against linear epitopes of Dsg3 (anti-Dsg3-L IgG).

Materials and Methods

Antibodies and Reagents

The 5H10 mouse monoclonal antibody against extracellular domains of Dsg3, anti-Dsg3 H-145 rabbit polyclonal antibodies raised against the cytoplasmic domain of Dsg3, H-290 rabbit antibodies against C-terminal residues 760-1046 of Dsg1, anti-pancytokeratin rabbit IgG and HRP-conjugated anti-rabbit and anti-mouse antibodies were from Santa Cruz Biotecnology (Santa Cruz, CA).

Texas Red- or FITC-conjugated anti-human, anti-mouse and anti-rabbit IgG antibodies were from DAKO (Dako Denmark A/S). Nitrocellulose filters were purchased from Invitrogen (Carlsbad, CA); ECL chemiluminescent immunodetection system and Hyperfilms were from Amersham (Buckinghamshire, U.K.). Cycloheximide (CX), protease inhibitors and cell culture reagents were from Sigma (St. Louis, MO), except keratinocyte growth medium (KGM), purchased from Gibco BRL (Gaithersburg, MD).

Sera, Total IgG Fractions, and Purified Anti-Dsg3-L IgG

Serum collection and purification of immunoglobulins were carried out following the experimental procedures detailed in chapter 2. Serum samples from patients with pemphigus foliaceus (PF, n=2) were a gentle gift from Prof. Vincenzo Ruocco.

Cell Cultures and Treatments

We cultured HaCaT cells as in chapter 2. At the time of the experiment, cells were seeded and grown to confluence on 35 mm Petri dishes. Eventually, cells were transferred to low calcium medium (Ca<0.1mM) supplemented with growth factors (KGM), according to the manufacturer's instructions.

For the analysis of desmoglein 3 half-life, cells were treated with 50 µg/ml CX to block protein synthesis and harvested at different time points.

Protein Extraction and Western Blot Analysis

Sequential protein extraction with C-HSU buffer was done according to our protocols, as described in chapter 3. For the analysis of desmoglein 3 half-life, cells were rinsed with complete PBS and scraped in PBS supplemented with protease inhibitors (phenylmethylsulfonylfluoride (PMSF) at 1 mM, 10 µg/ml leupeptin and 5 µg/ml aprotinin).

Pellets (800 x g for 10 minutes) with equivalent cell numbers (5×10^5) were resuspended in Laemmli sample buffer and loaded onto an 8% SDS-PAGE after heating for 5 min at 95°C. Proteins were transferred overnight onto nitrocellulose membranes at 20 V. Blocked membranes were incubated for 1 h with the primary antibody (1:1000) and then with specie-specific HRP-conjugated IgG (1:10000) as secondary antibody.

Bound antibodies were detected by ECL chemiluminescent immunodetection system. To ascertain that blots were loaded with equal amounts of protein lysates, filters were also incubated with a polyclonal antibody against β-actin protein. Band intensity was quantified by scanning films with the Molecular Analysis Software (Bio-Rad, Richmond, CA).

Immunoprecipitation

Pelleted cells from a 35 mm wells were suspended in immunoprecipitation buffer (50mM Tris-HCl, pH 7.5, 150 mM NaCl, 0.5% Nonidet P-40, 1 mM DTT, 1 mM PMSF) and centrifuged for 30 min at 16,000 g; 300 μl supernatants were incubated for 1 hour with PV serum 1:1, 20 μl anti-Dsg3 H-145 polyclonal antibodies or H-290 antibodies against Dsg1, after which 15 μl of protein A-Sepharose was added for two hours.

After centrifugation at 2,300 g for 10 min, beads containing antigen-antibody complexes were washed as described elsewhere to increase the efficiency of immunoprecipitation [114] and Western blotting was performed as detailed above.

For the immunoreactivity assay, IgG from 300 μl of PV serum were first precipitated with protein A-Sepharose at 16,000 g and PV-IgG-depleted serum was discarded. Proteins were extracted using low calcium immunoprecipitation (LCI) buffer (10 mM Tris-HCl, 5 mM EDTA, 0.5% Nonidet P-40, 1 mM DTT, 1 mM PMSF); then 600 μl supernatant was added to PV-IgG or 40 μl 5H10 anti-Dsg3 IgG for 2 hours and immunoprecipitation was continued as described above.

Standard and Semiquantitative Living-Cell Immunofluorescence (LCIF) Microscopy

Cells were grown on glass coverslips and incubated in the presence or absence of normal or PV complement-inactivated sera, with or without CX.

If necessary to improve the analysis, LCIF was used and semiquantitative results of fluorescence were taken, as detailed in chapter 3.

Results

a. Changes in Dsg3 turn-over and assembly

Pemphigus Serum Induces Reduction of Dsg3 Half-Life

To appreciate changes in Dsg3 half-life after exposure to PV and normal sera, we first assessed half-life of Dsg3 in keratinocytes cultured in normal conditions (DMEM + 10% FBS). Thus, cells were treated with 50 µg/ml CX and harvested at different time points afterward for the preparation of cell lysates. Dsg3 from cells grown in normal conditions showed a $t_{1/2}$ of about 24h (Figure 1. (a, b) *CX*), similar to that observed in HaCaT exposed to normal serum (not shown). When serum from PV patients was added together with CX, no relevant changes in Dsg3 half-life ($t_{1/2}$ ~23h) were revealed compared with controls, although after 24 hours the absolute amount dropped to about 20%, versus 50% of controls (*CX*), of the starting values (Figure 1. (a, b) *CX+PV*). However, pretreatment with PV serum 12 h before the addition of CX determined a reduction of Dsg3 half-life to ~18 hours (Figure 1. (a, b), *prePV+CX*), while cells pretreated with normal serum keep values of about 24 hours (not shown).

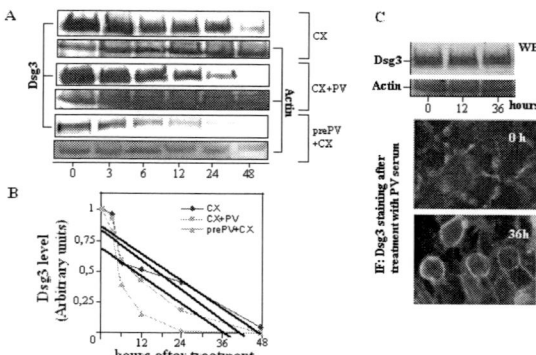

Figure 1. Treatments with sera and/or CX were conducted as described in the text. The level of Dsg3 was analyzed by using Western blot (**a**), quantified and normalized by measuring the density of Dsg3 and β-actin signals, and plotted using Microsoft Excel (**b**). Formulas for calculating t1/2 are: $Y_{CX} = -0.0181X + 0.865$; $Y_{CX+PV} = -0.0186X + 0.844$; $Y_{prePV+CX} = -0.0183X + 0.6675$. Straight lines were realized by considering the main values of three independent experiments. (**C**) Dsg3 levels by Western blot and immunofluorescence of HaCat cells within 36 h of treatment with 25% PV serum. Experiments shown in this figure were conducted using PV1 and C1 sera.

To exclude that changes observed by pretreating cells were related to a longer exposure to PV serum, we investigated the total amount of Dsg3 in response to sera along a 36 h period. Western blot and immunofluorescence analyses revealed that PV sera did not cause changes in the cellular amount of Dsg3 within 36 h, although cells became to round up (Figure 1(c)).

Thus, we considered the reduction of Dsg3 half-life as an effect of treating cells with PV sera before the addition of CX. It is reasonable that this finding is related to the ability of PV autoantibodies to bind newly synthesized Dsg3 that reached cell surface in the first 12 hours (i.e. before stopping protein synthesis) and have not yet established transinteraction.

PV IgG do Not Induce an Immediate Disruption of Assembled Desmosomes

To address whether serum PV IgG are able to dismantle desmosomal complexes, we stopped protein synthesis with CX to prevent formation of new desmosomes and then incubated cells with 25% PV sera. Immunofluorescence analysis showed PV IgG at sites of cell-cell contact, identified as punctate staining between adjacent cells, 24h after treatment (Figure 2 (a, b)). This finding suggests that PV autoantibodies are not able to disrupt desmosomal adhesion when stable contacts are done. Preincubation (12 hours) with PV serum, however, determined a decrease of PV IgG staining at desmosomal areas; indeed, fluorescence was revealed as a linear pattern all around cell borders (Figure 2. (a, c)).

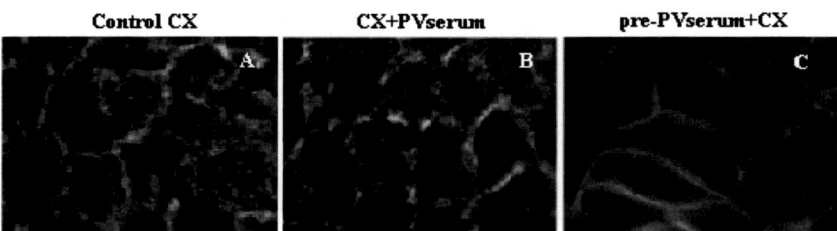

Figure 2. Immunofluorescence showing PV-IgG distributon on keratinocytes' surface. (a, b) FITC is localized in a punctate pattern within cell-cell contact areas. (C) In cells treated with PV serum 24 h before the addition of CX, PV-IgG described a diffuse, linear outline, on the entire cell surface. Figure is representative of independent experiments carried out with PV1-3 and C1-3 sera.

Thus, pemphigus serum is likely to perturb the stability of desmosomes by binding non-clustered Dsg3 before they have established interconnections with adjacent cells. Conversely, PV IgG do not deplete Dsg3 from adhesion sites nor disrupt preexisting desmosomes through direct interferences.

PV IgG-Bound Dsg3 is Not Early Internalized but Does Not Form Desmosomes

To understand whether Dsg3, when bound to PV IgG, is recruited at the sites of cell-cell contact to become assembled into desmosomes, we cultured keratinocytes in low calcium medium ($Ca^{2+}<0,1mM$). These culture conditions lead to a rapid loss of desmosomal adhesion by splitting such structures into desmosomal halves.

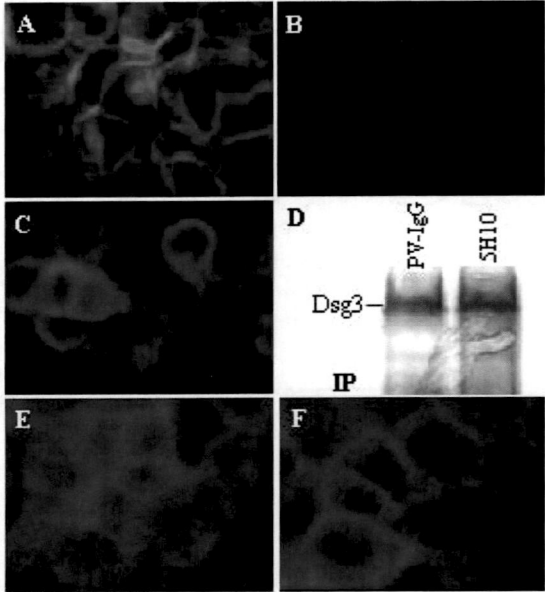

Figure 3. (a, b) The double-staining showed that FITC-positive (PV-IgG) sites also were stained with Texas Red (Dsg3); both PV-IgG and monoclonal 5H10 antibody were able to recognize (a,c) and immunoprecipitate (D) Dsg3 in low calcium conditions. PV-IgG were still labelled on keratinocytes' surface 9 (E) and 18 (F) hours after removing serum and switching cells to 0.9 mM Ca++. Figure is representative of independent experiments conducted with PV1-3 and C1-3 sera.

Although a loss of Dsg3 antigenicity after calcium depletion has been reported [121], we found that in our low calcium cell system PV IgG co-localize with, and are able to immunoprecipitate, Dsg3 (Figure 4. (a-d)).

Thus, the desmosome-deficient cells were exposed for 1h to 25% PV or normal serum, then media were changed and cultures switched to high calcium conditions to allow formation of stable desmosomes. As shown by immunofluorescence experiments, PV IgG localized at cell borders, suggesting that PV IgG-Dsg3 complexes were not markedly internalized within 18 hours after binding to PV autoantibodies (Figure 4. (e, f)).

To further investigate the effect of PV serum on cells forming *de novo* desmosomes, we trypsinized cells and, after removal of trypsin, plated them in presence of PV serum (25% final concentration). Within 12 h, cells became to aggregate and establish transinteraction, as revealed by an intense punctate staining of Dsg1 at sites of cell-cell contact (Figure 4. (c)). However, Dsg3 and PV IgG did not markedly enter the desmosomal pool, since both co-localized in a linear pattern (Figure 5. (a, b)).

After 36 h, desmosomes were no longer labelled on cell surface through Dsg1 and Dsg3 staining, suggesting that cell-cell contacts had been disrupted. Taken together, our data demonstrate that PV IgG do not cause a rapid disappearance of Dsg3 from cell surface but, when bound to non-desmosomal Dsg3, PV IgG prevent a stable assembly of Dsg3 into adhesion areas.

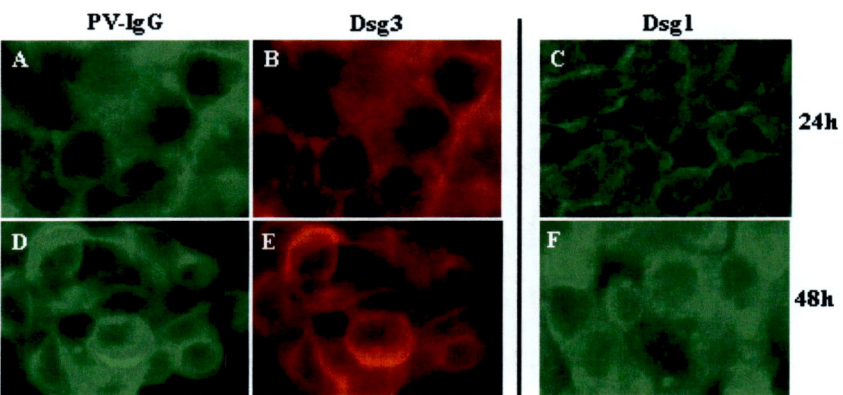

Figure 4. As revealed by double-staining immunofluorescence, Dsg3 bound to PV-IgG is almost absent in new formed desmosomes containing Dsg1 (punctate spots) after 24 hours of growth in presence of 25% PV serum (A-C). After 48 hours, cellular transinteraction were lacking (D-F), although Dsg still localized on cell borders. Figure is representative of independent experiments carried out with PV1-3 and C1-3 sera.

b. Modifications of Dsg1 expression and assembly

Anti-Dsg1 IgG-Containing Sera Induce Internalization of Dsg1 but Not Its Early Depletion from Desmosomes

To study the subcellular distribution of antibody-targeted Dsg1, we incubated HaCaT cells with PV (n=3), PF (n=2), PF-like (n=2) and control (n=2) sera. Cells exposed to H44211M IgG (PF-like serum) displayed a marked cytoplasmic trafficking of Dsg1, as revealed by the intense punctuate intracellular staining 6h after treatment (Figure 5. (d, e)).

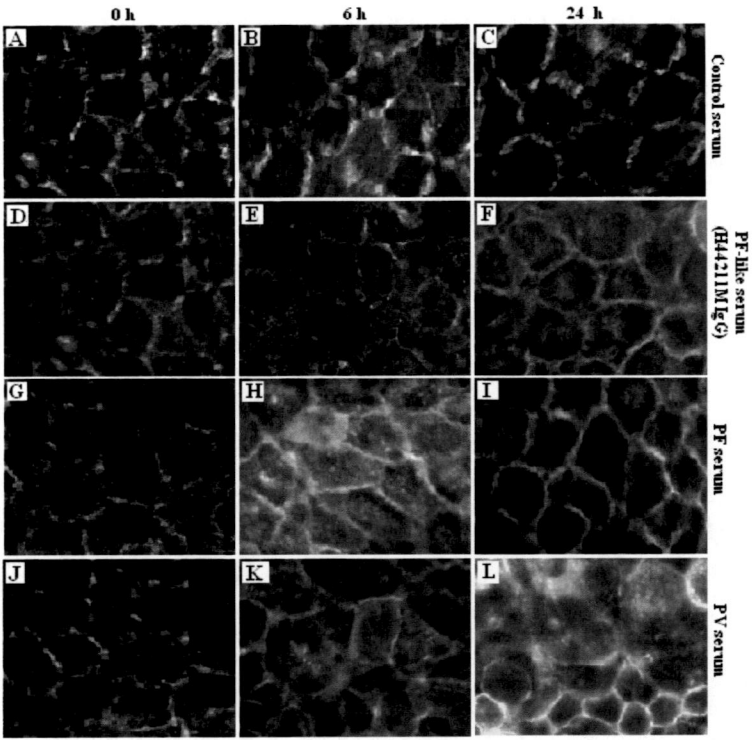

Figure 5. Internalization of antibody-targeted Dsg1. Sera from anti-Dsg1 IgG-containing sera induce internalization of Dsg1, as revealed by marked intracellular punctuate fluorescence within 6 hours of treatment (e,h,m). After 24 hours, Dsg1 was still present in aggregated clusters on surface of cells treated with PF and PF-like sera (e,i), whereas cells exposed to PV serum displayed a linear pattern of fluorescence along cell surface (n). See text for comments. Figures are representative of duplicate experiments carried out with sera of different patients.

After 24 h of exposure to PF-like serum, Dsg1 was still present on cell surface as punctuate clusters, referred to desmosomes, suggesting that H44211M IgG did not induce depletion of Dsg1 from sites of cell-cell adhesion (Figure 5. (f)). In keratinocytes incubated with pemphigus (PV and PF) serum for 6 h, Dsg1 was found redistributed within the intracellular compartment, being labelled at sites of cell-cell adhesion as well (Figure 5. (h,m)). However, PV serum exercised more dramatic effects on desmosomes, since punctuate staining of Dsg1 was grossly reduced 24 h after treatment, whereas PF serum did not induce marked changes on peripheral distribution of Dsg1 within 24 h (Figure 5. (i, n)); indeed, in cells exposed to PF serum, FITC fluorescence was distributed both in desmosomal (punctuate) and non-desmosomal areas, the latter revealed as a linear pattern over the entire cell surface (Figure 5. (i)). Taken together, these data suggest that binding of anti-Dsg1 antibodies to Dsg1 induces its internalization.

PF and PF-Like Autoantibodies Mobilize Prevalently Non-Clustered Dsg1

Immunofluorescence analysis showed PF-IgG at sites of cell-cell contact 24h after treatment (not shown). At time time, Dsg1 was still present into desmosomes (Figure 5. (c)). However, after exposure to PF serum, Dsg1 staining along non desmosomal areas was reduced (Figure 5. (b, c)). In the same conditions, Dsg3 labelling did not result affected by exposure to anti-Dsg1 IgG, providing strong evidence that redistribution of fluorescence was a Dsg1-specific phenomenon. Taken together, these findings suggest that PF autoantibodies are not able to directly disrupt Dsg1-containing adhesion complexes nor cause depletion of Dsg1 from desmosomes when stable contacts are done, but they just trigger internalization of unassembled, non-clustered, Dsg1.

Changes in Dsg1 Synthesis in Response to Anti-Dsg1 Antibodies

To test whether Dsg1 was depleted from the membrane fraction (including the newly synthesized pool) in response to anti-Dsg1 IgG, changes in Dsg1 synthesis were investigated by evaluating the Triton X-100 soluble (membrane) pool of protein from cells exposed to PV (n=3), PF (n=2) and PF-like (n=2) sera.

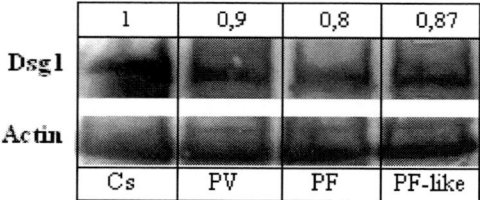

Figure 6. Western blot analysis of the membrane fraction of proteins. Anti-Dsg1 IgG-containing sera, but not control serum (Cs), determined reduction of the Triton X-100 soluble pool of Dsg1. Numbers represent the relative main values of Dsg1 levels (control serum =1) after normalization with β-actin, obtained from three independent experiments.

Western blot analysis revealed that the amount of the membrane fraction of Dsg1 decreased from 10 to 20% in cells exposed to anti-Dsg1 IgG-containing sera for 48h (Figure 6). These data demonstrate that PF autoantibodies decrease the rate of synthesis of Dsg1 in keratinocytes.

c. Processing of Dsg3 during acantholysis

Cleavage of Dsg3 in Keratinocytes Exposed to PV Serum

To elucidate the fate of Dsg3 in our *in vitro* model of PV (chapter 2), we carried out a time-course study and then investigated Dsg3 content in cell lysates through Western blotting. The amount of Dsg3 in keratinocytes decreased by approximately 75% along the 48-h-incubation with PV serum (Figure 7. (a)). Interestingly, a fragmentation product with apparent molecular mass of about 60 kDa (Figure 7. (a) *arrowhead*) reacting with the 5H10 monoclonal antibody against Dsg3 was detectable in detergent extracts by 3 hours after stimulation. Neither changes in full-length Dsg3 nor fragmentation products were detected in cell lysates from keratinocytes cultured in sera of healthy subjects (not shown). Densitometry values showed that time-dependent depletion of full-length Dsg3 paralleled with increase in signal intensity of the 60-kDa fragment (named fragment 1). Analysis of cell lysates with the H-145 antibody against the cytoplasmic domain of Dsg3 revealed that a band with apparent molecular mass of about 70 kDa, which was also detectable in normal conditions on lower levels, underwent biphasic increase of expression in lysates from PV-treated cells (Figure 7. (d)). Given that the molecular mass of the extracellular domain of Dsg3 is about 75 kDa, the proteolytic fragment would be expected to be shed in the culture supernatant. However, Western blotting of SFCM failed to show any reactivity against Dsg3 (not shown). Thus, we reasoned that cleavage of Dsg3 occurred intracellularly, leading to the formation of two proteolytic products of about 60-65 kDa (fragment 1) and 65-70 kDa (fragment 2).

Depletion of Dsg3 and Its Localization during Acantholysis by Semiquantitative LCIF

Expression and subcellular localization of Dsg3 in HaCaT cells exposed to PV sera were then investigated by semiquantitative LCIF. This technique has been recently demonstrated to be an approachable method to ameliorate the study of PV pathophysiology and morphological changes of keratinocytes [115]. PV serum-stimulated cells underwent progressive cell-cell detachment within 48 h (Figure 7. (b,c,f)).

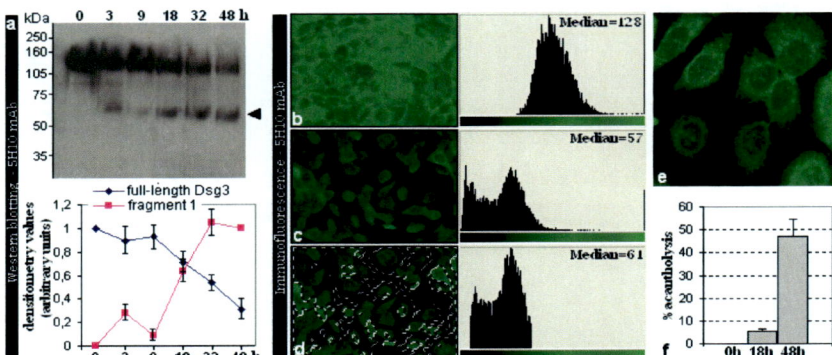

Figure 7. Cell lysates from time-course experiments were subjected to Western blotting against the 5H10 monoclonal antibody. Densitometry values were calculated after normalization with β-actin protein (a). Keratinocytes were exposed to normal (b) or PV serum (c) and then Dsg3 content was quantified by semiquantitative immunofluorescence (graphics of the right of panels express the median of green/FITC fluorescence intensity). In panel (d), fluorescence was quantified after subtracting black areas. Ten field of different photograms were used to calculate the mean values of acantholysis (f). Higher magnification photogram of Dsg3 staining in keratinocytes treated with PV serum for 24 h (e).

Concomitantly, the overall intensity of green (FITC) fluorescence that associated with both 5H10 (Figure 7. (b-d)) and H-145 (Figure 8. (b), *histogram*) antibodies was markedly reduced along the 48-h incubation time. In particular, Dsg3 staining was virtually abrogated from cell surface (Figure 7. (e) and 8. (b)). Consistently, the reduction of FITC fluorescence associated to cell periphery was concomitant with a diffuse staining of Dsg3 within the cytosol (Figure 7. (e)). Interestingly, intracellular domain of Dsg3 localized within the intracellular compartment as well, but it displayed robust accumulation around the perinuclear area (Figure 7. (b), *48h*). Thus, the two fragments localized in different subcellular areas, suggesting that they were physically distinct. To exclude these data to be biased by the presence of dark surfaces corresponding to the areas of intercellular detachment, we subtracted such a background and then calculated the intensity of green fluorescence. Within 48 hrs after exposure to PV sera, labelling of extracellular domain of Dsg3 was reduced of about 50% in comparison with control (Figure 7. (c)).

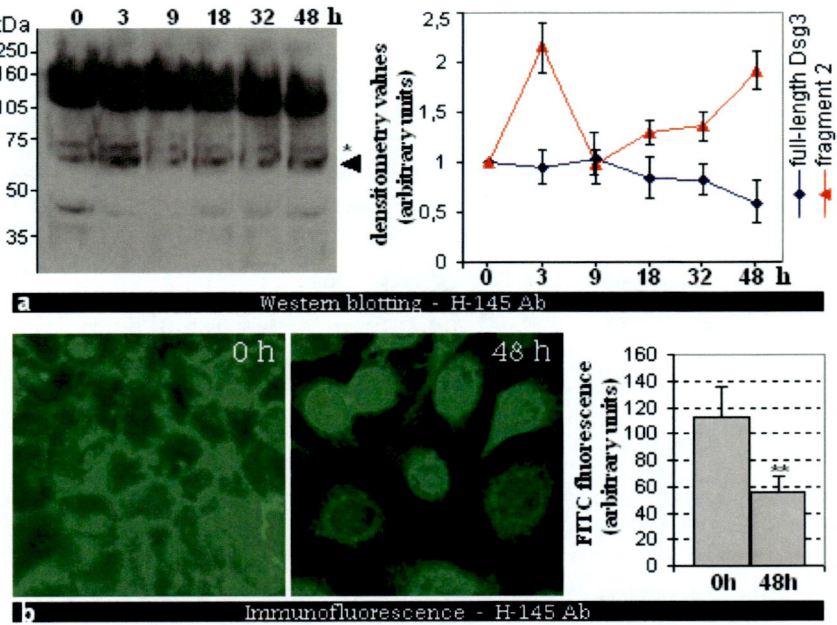

Figure 8. Keratinocytes were incubated with whole PV serum. The amount of Dsg3 along a 48-h time period was estima-ted by Western blotting (a) and semi-quantitative LCIF microscopy (b) by using the H-145 antibody against the cytoplasmic region of Dsg3. The band marked with an asterisk represents an unidentified and unspecific band. ** $p<0.01$.

This finding associated with formation of gross intercellular gaps (Figure 7. (b) and 8. (b) along with a marked reduction of adhesion strength among keratinocytes (not shown). Collectively, these findings strongly suggest that Dsg3 undergoes intracellular cleavage in cells exposed to PV serum.

d. Role of anti-Dsg3-L IgG in depleting Dsg3 from acantholytic cells

Depletion of Dsg3 by PV Serum and IgG Fractions

Depletion of Dsg3 from cells treated with anti-Dsg3 IgG has been recently reported [13]. Expression of Dsg3 in HaCaT cells exposed to PV1 serum, PV IgG, or anti-Dsg3-L IgG was initially investigated by semi-quantitative LCIF. This technique has been demonstrated by our group to be an approachable method to ameliorate the study of PV pathophysiology and the morphological changes of keratinocytes. In fact, living cell microscopy allows to avoid antigen distortion due to cell manipulation. Furthermore, evaluation of green (FITC) fluorescence by standard softwares allows to obtain semi-quantitative results of protein levels [116]. In pilot experiments, we found that keratinocytes exposed to PV1 serum underwent progressive cell-cell detachment by 12-24 h after treatment (Figure 9. (b)). Concomitantly, the overall intensity of green (FITC) fluorescence that associated with H-145 antibody was markedly reduced along the 24h incubation time (Figure 9. (e)). In particular, Dsg3 staining was virtually abrogated from cell surface (Figure 9. (b)). PV IgG-treated keratinocytes exhibited acantholytic features as well (Figure 9. (d)), although the amount of Dsg3 detected by the H-145 Ab did not decrease accordingly (Figure 9.(e)). PV2 and PV3 sera showed similar effects (Figure 9. (e)). Surprisingly, anti-Dsg3-L IgG failed to affect Dsg3 levels (Figure 9. (c, e)). Thus, we concluded that, although PV sera and PV IgG were pathogenic *in vitro*, their anti-Dsg3-L IgG fraction was not.

High-Dose Anti-Dsg3-L Can Induce Acantholysis and Reduction of Dsg3 Levels

We subsequently tested the pathogenicity of anti-Dsg3-L IgG on higher concentrations. After assessing optimal conditions, we diluted the purified antibodies in KAD medium at the final concentration of 1 µg/ml. Under these conditions, keratinocytes showed increased rates of dissociation (Figure 10. (a,b)), alterations in morphology, and cell-cell detachment (Figure 10. (c, d)).

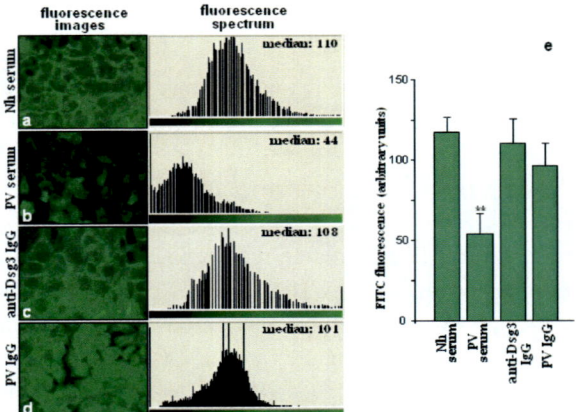

Figure 9. Results of semiquantitative fluorescence against Dsg3 in keratinocytes exposed to whole Nh1 serum (a), PV1 serum (b), 80 ng/ml anti-Dsg3 IgG (c), or 0.5 mg/ml PV IgG (d). Graphics of fluorescence spectrum express the median of green/FITC-fluorescence intensity. Results of at least two independent experiments with C1-2 and PV1-2 sera, and purified IgG were recorded and processed for statistical analysis (e). ** $p<0.01$.

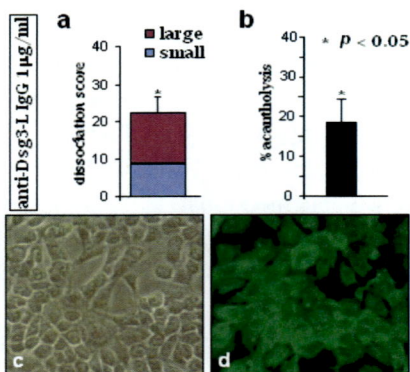

Figure 10. Dispase-based assay (a) and morphometric analysis of acantholysis (b) were carried out as detailed in materials and methods on keratinocytes incubated for 24 hours with 1 μg/ml anti-Dsg3 IgG. Morphology of cells after 24-h-incubation was recorded by phase contrast microscopy (c) and immunofluorescence with H-145 Ab (d).

In order to obtain comparable data, we then carried out additional experiments in accordance to previously published procedures [119]. Thus, keratinocytes were exposed to 2 ml whole PV sera (PV1-3), 0.5 mg PV IgG (pooled from PV1-3), or 1 µg/ml anti-Dsg3-L IgG (pooled from PV1-3) for 30 minutes, 24 and 48 hours.

Under these experimental conditions, semi-quantitative analysis of fluorescence revealed reduction of Dsg3 levels after both serum and IgG treatments (Figure 11). With these time points, the earliest significant changes occurred after 24-h incubation with whole PV serum ($p<0.05$).

In the presence of 1 µg/ml anti-Dsg3-L IgG, cell content of Dsg3 decreased of about 20% ($p<0.05$) in 48 h, whereas Dsg3 was approximately 30% less then control values ($p<0.01$) in cells exposed to 0.5 mg/ml PV IgG. About 60% Dsg3 was depleted from keratinocytes treated with whole PV sera for 48 h ($p<0.001$) (Figure 11).

Thus, the main result of these set of experiments was that anti-Dsg3 IgG against non-conformational epitopes of Dsg3 can induce alterations in keratinocytes in a dose- and time-dependent manner.

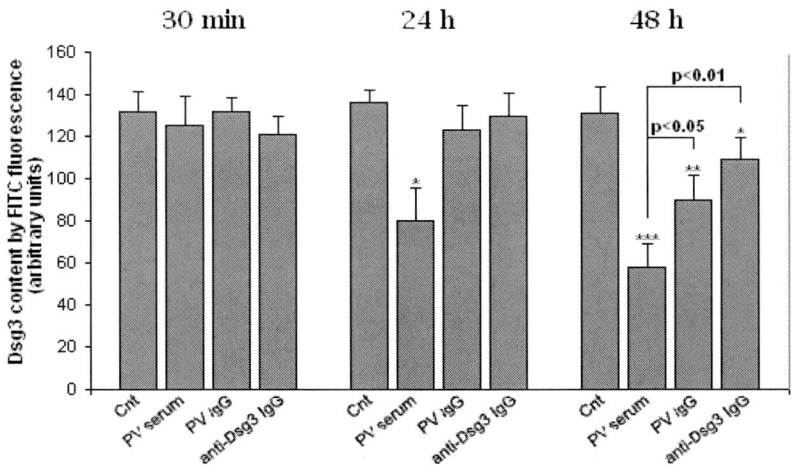

Figure 11. Cells were treated as shown (PV serum, 1µg/ml anti-Dsg3 IgG, 0.5 mg/ml PV IgG, or left untreated) and the amount of Dsg3 was quantified by living cell immunofluorescence (LCIF) microscopy by using the H-145 antibody against the cytoplasmic region of Dsg3. Ten fields of triplicate immunofluorescence photograms were used to calculate the mean values for Cnt, anti-Dsg3 IgG, and PV IgG. For evaluation of PV serum, results of two independent experiments carried out with PV1, PV2 and PV3 sera were considered.

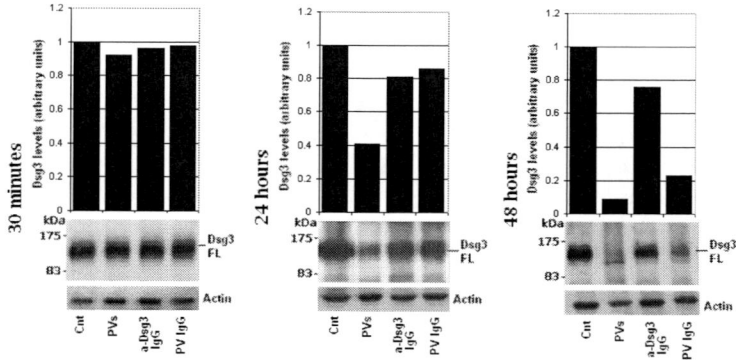

Figure 12. Cells Western blot analysis of total cell lysates (60 μg) from keratinocytes cultured for 30 minutes (a), 24 hours (b), or 48 hours (c), in the presence of PV2 serum (PVs), anti-Dsg3-L IgG at 1μg/ml (a-Dsg3 IgG), PV IgG (0.5 mg/ml), or left untreated (Cnt). The immunoblots were probed by using the H-145 antibody against Dsg3 or a polyclonal antibody against β-actin. Relative protein densities of full-length (FL) Dsg3 (130-140 kDa) were determined (histograms). Data reported here are representative of three independent experiments.

Next, Dsg3 protein levels were assessed by Western blotting of whole cell lysates. Early depletion of Dsg3 (30 min) was not found (Fiure 12. (a)). However, PV sera decreased the content of full-length Dsg3 in cell lysates by 24 h (Figure 12. (b)), and a dramatic reduction of full-length Dsg3 levels (91%) was observed within 48h after treatment (Figure 12. (c)). Keratinocytes treated with PV IgG or anti-Dsg3-L IgG for 24 h in both cases expressed about 80% Dsg3 (~20% depletion) in comparison with untreated controls (Figure 12. (b)). It should be noted, however, that the depleting activity of PV IgG reached ~70% after 48h, whereas at this time point keratinocytes treated with anti-Dsg3-L IgG retained 76% Dsg3 (24% depletion).

Taken together, the data from Dsg3-depletion assays provide evidence that anti-Dsg3-L IgG impact Dsg3 expression levels to a lesser extent than PV sera/IgG and solely when used on high concentration.

Discussion

a. Changes in Dsg3 turn-over and assembly

In the present section, we have demonstrated that an effect of PV serum is the reduction of Dsg3 half-life in keratinocytes. This finding could be related to the ability of PV autoantibodies to interfere with the stability of non-desmosomal Dsg3 but not of assembled desmosomes. Furthermore, binding of PV IgG to Dsg3 perturbs its recruitment at sites of intercellular contact and subsequent assembly into desmosomes.

Regulation of cell-cell adhesion appears to be a complex and finely orchestrated mechanism. Although autoantibodies against Dsg3 have been demonstrated to cause defects of intercellular adhesion [15, 18, 99], it remains unclear whether an impaired function of Dsg3 is sufficient to disrupt epithelial integrity. Indeed, the stability of intercellular junctions also relies on desmocollins and E-cadherin [122]. In PV patients, the finding of detectable titres of anti-ICS antibody not always associates with clinical manifestations of pemphigus and, however, blisters appear only in some areas of the body [60, 123]. Rather, PV IgG are likely to interfere with the delicate equilibrium underlying the maintenance of stable intercellular contacts. Our study demonstrates for what we believe is the first time that PV serum may induce acantholytic changes by reducing Dsg3 half-life and perturbing a stable assembly of Dsg3 into desmosomes. Furthermore, our evidence suggests that PV IgG do not cause desmosomal split, as instead has been previously reported in a mouse model of PV [124]. However, the PV IgG-decorated split-desmosomes described by Authors could be half-desmosomes-like clusters before their integration into stable complexes and not the result of desmosomal disruption.

The results of this study are in agreement with a view of the acantholysis as a well coordinate phenomenon in which a plethora of cell signals participates. One of the key points may be the reduction of Dsg3 half-life reported here. We favour the hypothesis that acantholysis takes place *in vivo* when cells become unable to maintain steady state levels of Dsg3. Our data also support the hypothesis that the defect of adhesion results from a perturbation of Dsg3 assembly into desmosomes. Nevertheless, it seems now clear that PV IgG can not induce disruption of already formed desmosomes.

In conclusion, this set of experiments have provided further insight into the mechanisms underlying epithelial blistering observed in pemphigus vulgaris. Reduction of Dsg3 half-life together with perturbation of its assembly into desmosomes may represent critical phenomena when cells result incapable of compensating this acquired deficit of adhesion and maintaining homeostasis.

b. Modifications of Dsg1 expression and assembly

Although is it well established that anti-Dsg1 antibodies from both PF and PV patients' sera are pathogenic [11], the fate of Dsg1 in response to such antibodies on the molecular and subcellular level remains substantially unexplored. In the present section, we have demonstrated that an effect of pemphigus sera is the internalization of Dsg1. This phenomenon is related to the action of Dsg1-targeting antibodies, since the redistribution of Dsg1 in the intracellular compartment occurs in response to a monoclonal anti-Dsg1 antibody as well. In particular, the data reported here support the idea that anti-Dsg1 antibodies found in PF serum induce the internalization of free, non-clustered pool of Dsg1 from cell surface, whereas they are not able to cause disruption of punctuate aggregates of Dsg1 referred to as desmosomes. The present is also the first demonstration that anti-Dsg1 antibodies from mucocutaneous PV sera exert similar effect on Dsg1 in comparison with those from PF sera. However, these phenomena did not associate with marked changes in Dsg1 expression, indicating that the activation of membrane trafficking machinery did not affect Dsg1 on a transcriptional level, as previously proposed to be the case of Dsg3 [42].

A question still open is whether anti-Dsg1 IgG induce acantholysis by steric hindrance of desmoglein interactions or triggering intracellular responses [118]. That is to say whether binding of IgG to Dsg1 induces its internalization, with subsequent disruption of the junctional complex, or whether the pathogenic antibody determines Dsg1-mediated signal transduction which drives desmosome disassembly as a final step of the cellular response, respectively. Data reported here uniquely provide evidence that in our experimental model anti-Dsg1 antibodies do not impair desmosome stability nor determine early depletion of Dsg1 from the adhesion sites in the first 6 h. Interestingly, the presence of anti-Dsg3 together with anti-Dsg1 antibodies seemed to accelerate the process of desmosome dissolution, since keratinocytes exposed to mucocutaneous PV serum did not exhibit the typical punctuate staining of Dsg1 on cell surface 24 h after treatment.

Another finding of our study is that antibodies against the extracellular domain of Dsg1 reproduce the same subcellular changes in Dsg1 distribution observed by using PF serum, making such antibodies useful to simulate the early cellular response to PF autoantibodies. Other pathogenic monoclonal antibodies have previously been tested for reproducing the experimental model of pemphigus vulgaris, such as PVMAB786 [99] and AK23 [125]. However, the H44211M used by us in the present study is the first anti-Dsg1 monoclonal antibody reported to be "pathogenic" in an *in vitro* model of PF.

In conclusion, here we defined the basic subcellular changes of keratinocyte Dsg1 occurring on *in vitro* models of Dsg1-targeting pemphigus types. Our results showed that anti-Dsg1 antibodies determined a marked internalization of Dsg1 without its early depletion from the adhesion sites.

c. Processing of Dsg3 during acantholysis

In this section, we report that pemphigus serum induces cleavage of Dsg3 in keratinocytes, with subsequent depletion of Dsg3 from cell lysates.

Dsg3 is important in maintaining epidermal adhesion [14]. Since its abrogation from keratinocytes parallel cell-cell detachment [42, 119], it is reasonable that Dsg3 processing and acantholysis are related phenomena. The main result of the set of experiments presented here is that depletion of full-length Dsg3 in PV is due to fragmentation processes affecting Dsg3. After stimulation of keratinocytes with PV sera, cleavage of Dsg3 occurs within 3 h leading to progressive formation of two fragmentation products with apparent molecular masses of about 60 kDa and 70 kDa (Fig.8). Consistent with the results of Western blotting, analysis of molecular masses of the two fragments suggests that cleavage does occur intracellularly. In fact, fragment 1 (60 kDa) reacted with the 5H10 mAb raised against the N-terminal residues 49-60 of Dsg3. Since the predicted mass of the extracellular portion of Dsg3 is 75 kDa, cleavage was supposed to affect the extracellular domain of Dsg3. Indeed, if cleavage of Dsg3 occurred extracellularly, fragment 1 was expected to be released into culture supernatant. Instead, we did not find any Dsg3 fragment in SFCM. Furthermore, given that the H-145 IgG raised against epitopes located within the cytoplasmic domain of Dsg3 did recognize a 70-kDa peptide (fragment 2), we concluded that fragmentation of Dsg3 resulted from a single cut. LCIF microscopy seemed to confirm our model. Indeed, immunofluorescence studies revealed 5H10 mAb to be localized diffusely within the cytoplasm of acantholytic cells, whereas H-145 accumulated around the nucleus. Since the two anti-Dsg3 antibodies did not colocalize, the intracellular labelling of Dsg3 is unlikely to result from internalization of full-length Dsg3. Furthermore, it should be noted that full-length Dsg3 almost disappeared from cell lysates 48h after treatment, whereas the respective amount of Dsg3 detected by LCIF was still robust. Taken together, these data account for a physical separation between the two tails of Dsg3 during acantholysis. They are also consistent with the hypothesis that the two fragmentation products are shed inside the cell.

Our findings provide an explanation of the abrogation of Dsg3 from the cell observed by other research groups. Indeed, Aoyama and Kitajima first reported depletion of Dsg3 from Triton-X-100 soluble pool of proteins after incubation of keratinocytes with PV sera, PV IgG [42], or anti-Dsg3 IgG [43]. This is in agreement with our present work wherein we have demonstrated reduction of Dsg3 half-life in response to PV serum. We currently don't know whether proteolysis of Dsg3 is part of an acantholytic program taking place after intracellular signals have been generated, of whether it is just the result of the action of anti-Dsg3 antibody. In the former, Dsg3 cleavage could be the result of apoptotic machinery; in the latter, Dsg3 fragmentation could depend on intracellular degradation which follows Dsg3 internalization. Further studies are needed to address these questions.

Collectively, our findings provide evidence that Dsg3 undergoes intracellular cleavage in response to PV serum. The subsequent depletion of Dsg3 from the cell may participate to the reduction of cell adhesion strength in pemphigus.

d. Role of anti-Dsg3-L IgG in Dsg3-depletion activity of PV serum and IgG

By means of Western blotting and semi-quantitative living cell immunofluorescence (LCIF) microscopy, here we reported that pemphigus serum and PV IgG can induce depletion of Dsg3 from keratinocytes, whereas the role of anti-Dsg3 IgG against linear epitopes of Dsg3 appeared to be more complex. Indeed, although sera of patients with PV are known to encompass pathogenic anti-Dsg3-L antibodies, the amount of such IgG purified from pathogenic volumes of whole PV sera did not induce acantholysis nor deplete keratinocytes of Dsg3 in our experimental model. However, the pathogenic potential of such polyclonal anti-Dsg3-L IgG was acquired at higher concentrations, corresponding to those found in 20-30-fold concentrated sera. Our data also suggest that depletion of Dsg3 may be a late event in acantholysis.

Reduction of Dsg3 levels from cell lysates has been reported after incubation of keratinocytes with PV sera, PV IgG, and anti-Dsg3 mAb. Accordingly, one can speculate that the ability of PV sera in depleting desmosomes of Dsg3 is related to the presence of pathogenic anti-Dsg3 IgG, including those targeting non-conformational epitopes of Dsg3 [120]. On the basis on the present data, however, the role of anti-Dsg3 IgG remains controversial. Among the key points to address in order to clarify this issue, the understanding of the "correct" amount of pathogenic antibodies and/or whole sera to be used is central [108]. With regard to this, recent work by Yasuo Kitajima demonstrated that anti-Dsg3 monoclonal antibodies of mouse origin exerted cumulative or synergistic effects in depleting keratinocytes and desmosomes of Dsg3. In particular, AK23 mAb at the concentration of 6.4 ng/ml was effective in reducing the amount of Dsg3 [119]. We found that 80 ng/ml purified anti-Dsg3 IgG pooled from 3 PV patients did not induce significant changes in HaCaT cells, whereas they depleted Dsg3 of about 20% when used at 1 μg/ml. These findings are consistent with the idea that the amount of anti-Dsg3-L IgG found in "pathogenic volumes" of PV sera are not able to induce acantholysis nor deplete Dsg3 from the cell.

The binding of PV IgG to their membrane targets is thought to affect primarily the Triton X-100-soluble, free membrane pool of Dsg3, whereas the delayed depletion of Dsg3 from Triton X-100-insoluble pools would reflect the subsequent abrogation of Dsg3 from desmosomes [42, 43]. However, recent paper by Waschke and colleagues reported that PV IgG increased Dsg3 in the triton-soluble fraction of cell lysates, indicating that the anchorage of Dsg3 to the cytoskeleton was reduced by pemphigus IgG [89]. They also demonstrated that Dsg3 levels were not substantially decreased in the cytoskeleton fractions after 24 h of incubation with PV IgG. To our knowledge, these discordant changes of Dsg3 levels in triton soluble pool of protein may be interpreted as either depletion of free membrane Dsg3 (if binding to non-desmosomal Dsg3 is predominant) or titration from the triton-insoluble to triton-soluble fraction (if binding to desmosomal Dsg3 with subsequent detachment from cytoskeleton is the pivotal event). Conflicting data reported above may also be explained by differences in the experimental conditions, including buffers for protein extraction and confluence of keratinocyte monolayers. However, given the discordance among the aforementioned findings, it is hard to draw conclusions about the physiopathological significance of the triton-soluble fraction of Dsg3. Therefore, in this study we have investigated the total amount of Dsg3 in cell lysates. By following this approach, we for the first time have gained insights into the role of IgG against linear epitopes of Dsg3 in the pathogenesis of PV.

The results reported here could also help to evaluate conflicting data in the literature on the action of PV IgG in vitro. Indeed, it was not entirely clear whether PV IgG deplete Dsg3 in confluent monolayers. By now depletion of Dsg3 has been only found by in monolayers of 40% confluence [119]. We found significant changes in Dsg3 expression induced by PV IgG in confluent keratinocytes. The differences in relative Dsg3 levels reported by means of either LCIF or Western blotting may be explained by the fact that fluorescence data reflect the presence in situ of fragmentation products and/or metabolic intermediates of Dsg3 in addition to the full-length protein. On the contrary, quantitation of band intensities on Western blots is based on the levels of full-length Dsg3 in cell lysates. Thus, the data presented by us unequivocally indicate effective depletion of Dsg3 by both whole PV serum and PV IgG. PV sera exhibited the highest depleting activity, which may be partially due to the participation of non-IgG serum factors such as FasL in acantholysis. Further studies will elucidate the actual contribution of cytokines and/or pro-apoptotic molecules in depleting Dsg3 from the cell.

Finally, it should be noted that comparison between data from morphometric/functional analyses and Western blotting/LCIF assays suggest that Dsg3 depletion is not required for acantholysis, rather it may represent its consequence. Indeed, 500 g/ml PV IgG or 1 g/ml anti-Dsg3-L IgG were able to induce acantholysis in keratinocyte monolayers within 24 h (Fig.9 and Fig.10, respectively), yet no substantial depletion of Dsg3 was observed either in situ (Fig.11) or in cell lysates (Fig.12b) during the same time period. Reduction of Dsg3 levels in fact seemed to be a late event in acantholysis. This is consistent with the hypothesis that disruption of desmosomes is not only a non-causal event in PV, but also represents a subsequent event which occurs when cells have already begun to shrink and detach [95].

Collectively, our findings provide evidence that Dsg3 undergoes depletion in keratinocytes exposed to PV serum and PV IgG, but this phenomenon does not seem to strictly correlate with the activity of anti-Dsg3-L IgG. In particular, depletion of Dsg3 from the cell occurs solely in response to high-dose anti-Dsg3-L IgG. These data suggest IgG against non-conformational epitopes of Dsg3 to play a minor role in depleting desmosomes of Dsg3. Furthermore, the results presented here support the hypothesis that depletion of Dsg3 occurs late in acantholysis.

e. Processing of Dsg3 during acantholysis

In this section, we report that pemphigus serum induces cleavage of Dsg3 in keratinocytes, with subsequent depletion of Dsg3 from cell lysates.

Dsg3 is important in maintaining epidermal adhesion [14]. Since its abrogation from keratinocytes parallel cell-cell detachment [42, 119], it is reasonable that Dsg3 processing and acantholysis are related phenomena. The main result of the set of experiments presented here is that depletion of full-length Dsg3 in PV is due to fragmentation processes affecting Dsg3. After stimulation of keratinocytes with PV sera, cleavage of Dsg3 occurs within 3 h leading to progressive formation of two fragmentation products with apparent molecular masses of about 60 kDa and 70 kDa (Figure 8). Consistent with the results of Western blotting, analysis of molecular masses of the two fragments suggests that cleavage does occur intracellularly. In fact, fragment 1 (60 kDa) reacted with the 5H10 mAb raised against the N-terminal residues 49-60 of Dsg3. Since the predicted mass of the extracellular portion of Dsg3 is 75 kDa, cleavage was supposed to affect the extracellular domain of Dsg3. Indeed, if cleavage of Dsg3 occurred extracellularly, fragment 1 was expected to be released into culture supernatant. Instead, we did not find any Dsg3 fragment in SFCM. Furthermore, given that the H-145 IgG raised against epitopes located within the cytoplasmic domain of Dsg3 did recognize a 70-kDa peptide (fragment 2), we concluded that fragmentation of Dsg3 resulted from a single cut. LCIF microscopy seemed to confirm our model. Indeed, immunofluorescence studies revealed 5H10 mAb to be localized diffusely within the cytoplasm of acantholytic cells, whereas H-145 accumulated around the nucleus. Since the two anti-Dsg3 antibodies did not colocalize, the intracellular labelling of Dsg3 is unlikely to result from internalization of full-length Dsg3. Furthermore, it should be noted that full-length Dsg3 almost disappeared from cell lysates 48h after treatment, whereas the respective amount of Dsg3 detected by LCIF was still robust. Taken together, these data account for a physical separation between the two tails of Dsg3 during acantholysis. They are also consistent with the hypothesis that the two fragmentation products are shed inside the cell.

Our findings provide an explanation of the abrogation of Dsg3 from the cell observed by other research groups. Indeed, Aoyama and Kitajima first reported depletion of Dsg3 from Triton-X-100 soluble pool of proteins after incubation of keratinocytes with PV sera, PV IgG [42], or anti-Dsg3 IgG [43]. This is in agreement with our present work wherein we have demonstrated reduction of Dsg3 half-life in response to PV serum. We currently don't know whether proteolysis of Dsg3 is part of an acantholytic program taking place after intracellular signals have been generated, of whether it is just the result of the action of anti-Dsg3 antibody. In the former, Dsg3 cleavage could be the result of apoptotic machinery; in the latter, Dsg3 fragmentation could depend on intracellular degradation which follows Dsg3 internalization. Further studies are needed to address these questions.

Collectively, our findings provide evidence that Dsg3 undergoes intracellular cleavage in response to PV serum. The subsequent depletion of Dsg3 from the cell may participate to the reduction of cell adhesion strength in pemphigus.

 f. Role of anti-Dsg3-L IgG in Dsg3-depletion activity of PV serum and IgG

By means of Western blotting and semi-quantitative living cell immunofluorescence (LCIF) microscopy, here we reported that pemphigus serum and PV IgG can induce depletion of Dsg3 from keratinocytes, whereas the role of anti-Dsg3 IgG against linear epitopes of Dsg3 appeared to be more complex. Indeed, although sera of patients with PV are known to encompass pathogenic anti-Dsg3-L antibodies, the amount of such IgG purified from pathogenic volumes of whole PV sera did not induce acantholysis nor deplete keratinocytes of Dsg3 in our experimental model. However, the pathogenic potential of such polyclonal anti-Dsg3-L IgG was acquired at higher concentrations, corresponding to those found in 20-30-fold concentrated sera. Our data also suggest that depletion of Dsg3 may be a late event in acantholysis.

Reduction of Dsg3 levels from cell lysates has been reported after incubation of keratinocytes with PV sera, PV IgG, and anti-Dsg3 mAb. Accordingly, one can speculate that the ability of PV sera in depleting desmosomes of Dsg3 is related to the presence of pathogenic anti-Dsg3 IgG, including those targeting non-conformational epitopes of Dsg3 [120]. On the basis on the present data, however, the role of anti-Dsg3 IgG remains controversial. Among the key points to address in order to clarify this issue, the understanding of the "correct" amount of pathogenic antibodies and/or whole sera to be used is central [108]. With regard to this, recent work by Yasuo Kitajima demonstrated that anti-Dsg3 monoclonal antibodies of mouse origin exerted cumulative or synergistic effects in depleting keratinocytes and desmosomes of Dsg3. In particular, AK23 mAb at the concentration of 6.4 ng/ml was effective in reducing the amount of Dsg3 [119]. We found that 80 ng/ml purified anti-Dsg3 IgG pooled from 3 PV patients did not induce significant changes in HaCaT cells, whereas they depleted Dsg3 of about 20% when used at 1µg/ml. These findings are consistent with the idea that the amount of anti-Dsg3-L IgG found in "pathogenic volumes" of PV sera are not able to induce acantholysis nor deplete Dsg3 from the cell.

The binding of PV IgG to their membrane targets is thought to affect primarily the Triton X-100-soluble, free membrane pool of Dsg3, whereas the delayed depletion of Dsg3 from Triton X-100-insoluble pools would reflect the subsequent abrogation of Dsg3 from desmosomes [42, 43]. However, recent paper by Waschke and colleagues reported that PV IgG increased Dsg3 in the triton-soluble fraction of cell lysates, indicating that the anchorage of Dsg3 to the cytoskeleton was reduced by pemphigus IgG [89]. They also demonstrated that Dsg3 levels were not substantially decreased in the cytoskeleton fractions after 24 h of incubation with PV IgG. To our knowledge, these discordant changes of Dsg3 levels in triton soluble pool of protein may be interpreted as either depletion of free membrane Dsg3 (if binding to non-desmosomal Dsg3 is predominant) or titration from the triton-insoluble to triton-soluble fraction (if binding to desmosomal Dsg3 with subsequent detachment from cytoskeleton is the pivotal event). Conflicting data reported above may also be explained by differences in the experimental conditions, including buffers for protein extraction and confluence of keratinocyte monolayers. However, given the discordance among the aforementioned findings, it is hard to draw conclusions about the physiopathological significance of the triton-soluble fraction of Dsg3. Therefore, in this study we have investigated the total amount of Dsg3 in cell lysates. By following this approach, we for the first time have gained insights into the role of IgG against linear epitopes of Dsg3 in the pathogenesis of PV.

The results reported here could also help to evaluate conflicting data in the literature on the action of PV IgG *in vitro*. Indeed, it was not entirely clear whether PV IgG deplete Dsg3 in confluent monolayers. By now depletion of Dsg3 has been only found by in monolayers of 40% confluence [119]. We found significant changes in Dsg3 expression induced by PV IgG in confluent keratinocytes. The differences in relative Dsg3 levels reported by means of either LCIF or Western blotting may be explained by the fact that fluorescence data reflect the presence *in situ* of fragmentation products and/or metabolic intermediates of Dsg3 in addition to the full-length protein. On the contrary, quantitation of band intensities on Western blots is based on the levels of full-length Dsg3 in cell lysates. Thus, the data presented by us unequivocally indicate effective depletion of Dsg3 by both whole PV serum and PV IgG. PV sera exhibited the highest depleting activity, which may be partially due to the participation of non-IgG serum factors such as FasL in acantholysis. Further studies will elucidate the actual contribution of cytokines and/or pro-apoptotic molecules in depleting Dsg3 from the cell.

Finally, it should be noted that comparison between data from morphometric/functional analyses and Western blotting/LCIF assays suggest that Dsg3 depletion is not required for acantholysis, rather it may represent its consequence. Indeed, 500 µg/ml PV IgG or 1 µg/ml anti-Dsg3-L IgG were able to induce acantholysis in keratinocyte monolayers within 24 h (Figure 9. and Figure 10, respectively), yet no substantial depletion of Dsg3 was observed either in situ (Figure 11) or in cell lysates (Figure 12. (b) during the same time period. Reduction of Dsg3 levels in fact seemed to be a late event in acantholysis. This is consistent with the hypothesis that disruption of desmosomes is not only a non-causal event in PV, but also represents a subsequent event which occurs when cells have already begun to shrink and detach [95].

Collectively, our findings provide evidence that Dsg3 undergoes depletion in keratinocytes exposed to PV serum and PV IgG, but this phenomenon does not seem to strictly correlate with the activity of anti-Dsg3-L IgG. In particular, depletion of Dsg3 from the cell occurs solely in response to high-dose anti-Dsg3-L IgG. These data suggest IgG against non-conformational epitopes of Dsg3 to play a minor role in depleting desmosomes of Dsg3. Furthermore, the results presented here support the hypothesis that depletion of Dsg3 occurs late in acantholysis.

Chapter 5

Role of Non-Desmoglein and Non-IgG Autoimmunity in PV

The pathogenesis of pemphigus vulgaris (PV) is currently traced back to the action of autoantibodies against antigens located within the intercellular substance (ICS) of keratinocytes, represented mainly by the desmosomal cadherin desmoglein 3 (Dsg3). Accordingly, titres of anti-ICS and anti-Dsg3 IgG are considered as major laboratory criteria to make diagnosis of PV. In this section, we used a non-conventional apparoach and demonstrated for the first time that a) PV IgG bind antigen(s) expressed on the surface of peripheral blood mononuclear cells (PBMC), and b) PV sera depleted of IgG can induce well-defined changes on keratinocyte morphology and metabolic activity.

The novel PBMC autoantigen is immunoprecipitated by PV IgG as a 130-kDa protein. However, western blot analysis of the immunocomplexes failed to show reactivity with anti-Dsg3 monoclonal and polyclonal antibodies. Taken together, our data provide strong evidence that PV autoimmunity targets a 130 kDa antigen other than Dsg3 on PBMC. This shifting from epidermis to blood cells may open new perspectives for a better understanding of pemphigus autoimmunity and more rational approaches to its treatment.

PV IgG-free sera determined marked alterations on cell shape, accompanied by partial loss of keratinocyte-keratinocyte interactions within 48 h after treatment. Furthermore, PV IgG-depleted sera caused a PERK-dependent reduction of cell viability together with a less sustained weakening of intercellular adhesion strength. Thus, in light of the above findings, loss of cell-cell adhesion in PV occurs as a result of the cooperating action of both IgG and non-IgG-mediated mechanisms.

These data have remarkable consequences on experimental models of PV and might open new "biological" approaches to its therapy. Thus, researchers are well advised that PV pathophysiology cannot be faithfully reproduced by leaving non-IgG serum factors out of consideration.

Introduction

Almost all patients with PV have pathogenic circulating IgG autoantibodies which bind to normal components of keratinocyte cell membrane belonging to the cadherin supergene family. Immunoblotting and immunoprecipitation studies demonstrated the autoantigen of PV as the 130-140 kDa desmoglein 3 (Dsg3) [10]. However, the catalogue of putative self antigens recognized by PV IgG include non-desmoglein molecules such as desmocollins, plakoglobin, and desmoplakin, all involved in regulating cell-cell adhesion of keratinocytes (reviewed in chapter 1). In addition to cell adhesion molecules, compelling evidence now attests to the role of IgG against keratinocyte cholinergic receptors in the disruption of cell-cell contacts leading keratinocytes to separate from one another [8, 25-27]. The binding of the autoantibodies to their targets generates a plethora of biological effects due, on one hand, to their direct interference with desmogleins' adhesive function and, on the other, to more complex events involving intracellular pathways that modify cell phosphorilation status, proteases activity or calcium metabolism, leading to loss of cell-cell adhesion (reviewed in ref. 57).

Recently, the discovery of a circulating 30 kDa fragment of desmoglein 3 (sDsg3) has moved the attention from tissue restricted epithelial Dsg3 to that found in serum [114]. Indeed, recognition of immunogenic epitopes of PV autoantigen may be crucial for the initiation and perpetuation of specific T and B cell responses, as well as for the induction of tolerance. In line with this concept, the availability of the self antigen represents a key point for immune function regulation. We have supposed that sDsg3 can stem from cleavage of keratinocyte Dsg3; however, the presence of full-length Dsg3 on blood cells has never been investigated. Hence, in this section, we first tried to assess whether PV antigens exist that are expressed by cells other than keratinocytes.

The second endpoint of the present chapter was to understand whether non-IgG factors take part in development of acantholysis. Although a critical role for autoantibodies in PV seems in fact undeniable, in recent years PV pathogenesis has been revisiting.

Recent studies have provided evidence that pemphigus acantholysis is related to a series of cytokines, such as IL-1α, TNF-α [28, 29], IL-6 [30] and IL-10 [31, 32]. Although it is not clear whether cytokines do play a pathogenic action, they could be critical in regulating the delicate equilibrium ensuring the maintenance of cell adhesion.

To investigate the role of serum factors other than IgG in PV pathogenesis, we examined the effects of IgG-depleted sera on keratinocyte monolayers. The results obtained in the present study raised intriguing perspectives, as they represent the first demonstration that PV sera can exercise relevant effects on keratinocyte shape and metabolic activity in absence of autoantibodies.

Materials and Methods

Antibodies and Reagents

The 5H10 mouse monoclonal antibody (mAb) recognizing the N-terminal residues 49-60 within the extracellular domain of Dsg3, anti-Dsg3 H-145 rabbit polyclonal antibodies raised against the cytoplasmic domain of Dsg3, H-290 rabbit antibodies against C-terminal residues 760-1046 of Dsg1 and HRP-conjugated anti-rabbit and anti-mouse antibodies were from Santa Cruz Biotecnology (Santa Cruz, CA). The H44211M mouse monoclonal antibody against the extracellular domain of Dsg1 [126] was from Biodesign International (Saco, MA).

The 5G11 mAb against the extracellular domain of Dsg3 was from Zymed Laboratories (Invitrogen immunodetection, San Francisco, CA), FITC-conjugated anti-human, anti-mouse and anti-rabbit IgG antibodies were from DAKO (Dako Denmark A/S). PVDF filters and RPMI were purchased from Invitrogen (Carlsbad, CA); ECL chemiluminescent immunodetection system and Hyperfilms were from Amersham (Buckinghamshire, U.K.). Protease inhibitors and all cell culture reagents, with the exception of RPMI, were from Sigma (St. Louis, MO).

Whether not otherwise stated, figures shown in the present study were obtained using PV1 and control 1 sera. Results were confirmed in independent experiments with PV2-4 sera.

Preparation of IgG-Free Sera and Igg Purification

Serum samples were incubated with appropriate amounts of Protein A-Sepharose microbeads (Sigma) for 2 hours, followed by centrifugation at 10,000 x g. The supernatant was transferred to a new tube and stored at -80°C as IgG-free serum.

Bound IgG were released from the beads with glycine 0.1 M and pH was rapidly adjusted by adding large volumes of TBS. IgG were then lyophilized and stored at -80°C. Alternatively, sera were filtered with 50 kDa cut-off filters (Biomax-50, Millipore). IgG-free sera obtained with the two methods were tested separately in pilot essays and found to exercise similar effects. Experiments shown in the present paper were realized by using 50 kDa-filtered PV1 serum. Results were confirmed by probing all sera in at least two independent experiments.

Cell Cultures, Treatments and siRNA transfections

HaCaT cells were maintained as dedailed in chapter 2.

Peripheral blood was collected from two healthy donors in heparinized tubes, transferred to polypropylene tubes and diluted with RPMI 1640 medium. PBMC were isolated using Ficoll HyPaque density gradient centrifugation.

Aliquots of 1 x 10^6 freshly isolated PBMC were washed with ice-cold PBS, pelleted at 800 x g and stored at -80°C until further analysis. PBMC were cultured *in vitro* in RPMI 1640 supplemented with non-essential amino acids and 10% FBS.

For siRNA experiments, see protocols reported in chapter 6.

Protein Extraction, Western Blotting, and Immunoprecipitation

Pooled cells were rinsed with complete PBS supplemented with protease inhibitors (phenylmethylsulfonylfluoride (PMSF) at 1 mM, 10 μg/ml leupeptin and 5 μg/ml aprotinin) and pellets (800 x g for 10 minutes) were resuspended in Triton buffer (50mM Tris-HCl, pH 7.5, 150 mM NaCl, 5 mM EDTA, 1% Triton X-100, 1 mM DTT, 1 mM PMSF).

Equal amounts of protein (60 μg per lane) were mixed with 4X Laemmli sample buffer and loaded onto an 8% SDS-PAGE after heating for 5 min at

95°C. Western blot analysis was carried out according to standard procedures (chapter 2).

Pelleted cells were suspended in immunoprecipitation buffer (50mM Tris-HCl, pH 7.5, 150 mM NaCl, 0.5% Nonidet P-40, 1 mM DTT, 1 mM PMSF) and centrifuged for 30 min at 16,000 g. Supernatants containing equal amounts of protein (300 µg) were precleared with 15 µl of protein A-Sepharose and then incubated for 1 hour with PV serum, after which 15 µl of protein A-Sepharose was added for two hours. After centrifugation at 2,300 g for 10 min, beads containing antigen-antibody complexes were washed as described elsewhere to increase the efficiency of immunoprecipitation [114] and Western blotting was performed as detailed above.

Gel Purification of 130 kDa Bands

For purification of both keratinocyte and PBMC 130 kDa band, the protein samples immunoprecipitated from cell lysates were loaded onto an 8% preparative polyacrylamide gel and separated at 100 V for two hours; a 5 mm-wide band, corresponding to the 133-kDa prestained marker, was excised and dehydrated in ACN; subsequently, gel containing the 130-kDa protein(s) was incubated for 2h at 37°C in bicarbonate elution buffer (50 mM ammonium bicarbonate, 0.1% SDS) after which a solution of isopropanol-formic acid was added to a final concentration of 45-5% (v/v) for 30 min at room temperature. The eluted proteins were lyophilized, and the SDS was removed by washings with cold 80% acetone.

Finally, for control studies, PV IgG were incubated with 1ml of gel pure 130-kDa protein(s) for 1 hour and than diluted in appropriate antibody solution and used for immunoblotting or immunofluorescence.

Immunofluorescence Microscopy

Keratinocytes were grown to confluence on glass coverslips in DMEM plus 10% FBS. Cultured PBMC were collected in 2 ml tubes and pelleted at 800 x g. Standard immunofluorescence microscopy and LCIF were performed as reported (chapter 2).

Metabolic activity Assay Using MTT

Assessment of the activity of living cells, based on mitochondrial function, was determined by the ability of cells to convert soluble MTT (3-(4,5-dimethylthiazol-2-yl)-2–5-diphenyltetrazolium bromide) into the insoluble purple formazan reaction product. HaCaT cells were plated on 12-well dishes and cultured with complete FAD until they reached confluence. Then, cells were treated with both control and PV (whole or IgG-free) sera (50% v/v) for 36 h.

During the last 4 h of incubation time, the media were replaced by MTT solution (10% v/v in DMEM without phenol red), 1 ml for each well. The MTT solution was then aspirated and formazan was dissolved by addition of 1 ml 0.1 N HCl. In all cases, cells were examined under phase-contrast microscope before application of MTT to visually assess the degree of cell death.

The absorbance of the supernatants was read at 570 nm wavelength. Percentage of cell viability (MTT conversion into purple formazan, in comparison with control values) indicates rates of mitochondrial respiration or activity of mitochondrial dehydrogenases.

Cell Dissociation Assay

Dispase-based cell dissociation assay was conducted as reported by us previously [127]. Briefly, confluent cells were exposed to 50% sera for 24-48 h, then media were removed and cells washed three times in PBS.

To release monolayers from substrate, HaCaT were incubated for 1h in 0.25% dispase. Epithelial sheets were transferred to 15 ml conical tubes containing 4 ml PBS and subjected to mechanical stress by turning tubes upside down 20 times. Cells were returned to Petri dishes and the degree of fragmentation was estimated by counting particles of more than 3mm.

Results

PBMC do not express desmoglein 1 and 3. To investigate whether PV antigens were expressed by PBMC, we carried out immunofluorescence studies with monoclonal antibodies against Dsg1 and Dsg3.

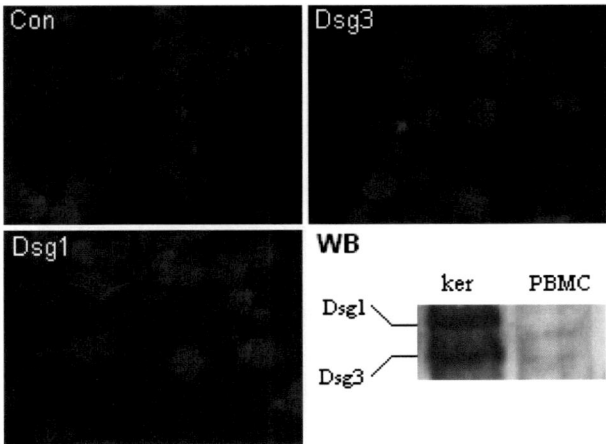

Figure 1. Immunofluorescence studies and Western blotting (WB) showed that PBMC lack Dsg1 and Dsg3. Anti-Dsg1 and anti-Dsg3 were first probed separately, then the results were summarized in the same blot by incubating PVDF filters with both antibodies. Keratinocyte lysates (ker) served as positive control. C, negative control PBMC obtained by using only FITC-conjugated anti-human antibodies. Figure is representative of three independent experiments.

Consistent with the assumption that blood cells do not assemble desmosomes, these desmosomal proteins were found to be undetectable on PBMC (Figure 1),. Slight green fluorescence was appreciated both in negative controls (Con) and PBMC probed for Dsg1 and Dsg3. This was likely to reflect the unspecific binding of FITC-conjugated secondary antibody on cell surface. Western blotting on cell lysates confirmed that PBMC expressed neither Dsg1 nor Dsg3 (Figure 1, WB).

PV IgG Immunoprecipitate a PBMC 130 kDa Protein Other than Dsg3

Since PV IgG bind antigens located in the epidermis, the immunoreactivity of PV sera is classically assessed by using keratinocyte extracts as antigen source. To test whether antigen(s) exist in blood cells that are recognized by PV sera, IgG of patients with PV were used to immunoprecipitate protein extracts from PBMC. Surprisingly, Ponceau staining of PVDF filters showed that PV IgG, but not normal IgG, immunoprecipitated a 130 kDa protein (Figure 2. (a, b)). By using combined immunoprecipitation-western blotting with PV IgG as primary antibody, the 130 kDa band was confirmed to be selectively recognized by IgG of patients with PV (Figure 2(c)). Furthermore, pre-incubation of PV IgG with the 130 kDa protein(s) purified from keratinocyte extracts strongly reduced the signal (Figure 2. (d)), suggesting that the novel PV antigen was expressed on both keratinocytes and PBMC.

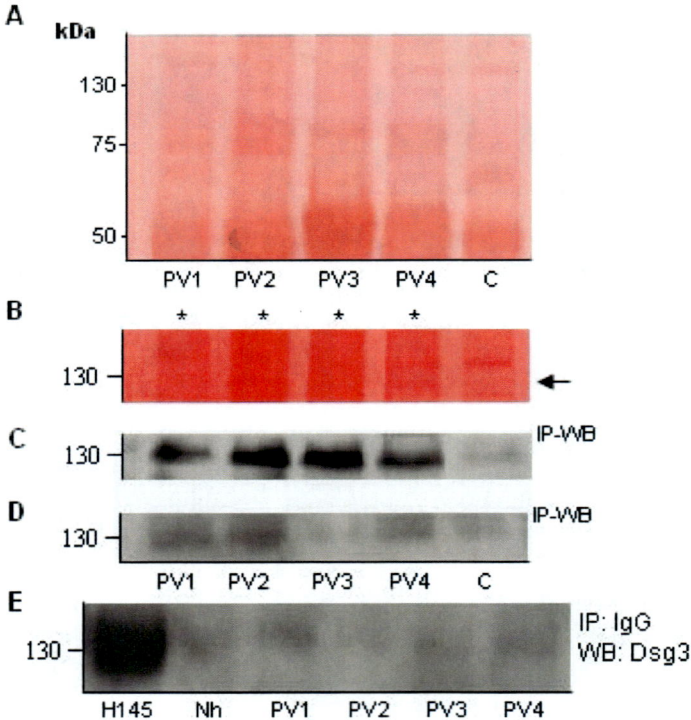

Figure 2. (a) Ponceau staining of PVDF membranes blotted with immunocomplexes shows a slight 130 kDa band immunoprecipitated by PV (n=4) but not control sera. (b) By enhancing contrast of the surface of interest (Adobe Photoshop), the 130 kDa band (arrow) clearly appeared in lanes 1-4 (PV sera, asterisks) but not in lane 5 (control). (c) Combined immunoprecipitation (IP)-western blotting (WB) with PV IgG demonstrated that IgG from PV sera recognized a 130 kDa protein. (d) Pre-incubation of PV IgG (primary antibody) with gel pure 130 kDa protein(s) from keratinocyte extracts strongly reduced the ability of PV IgG to bind the 130 kDa PBMC antigen. (e) Immunoprecipitation of keratinocyte extracts with H-145 anti-Dsg3 (positive control), Nh or PV IgG followed by WB against Dsg3 revealed that immunocomplexes other than positive control did not contain Dsg3. Results were confirmed at least in two experiment carried out independently.

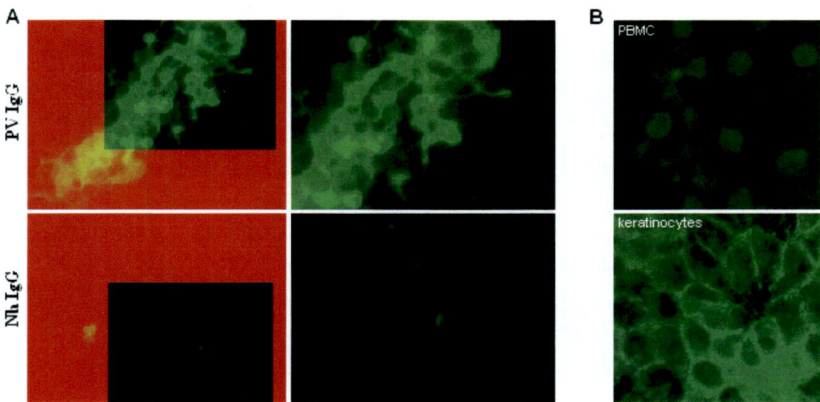

Figure 3. (a) PBMC were fixed and permeabilized in paraformaldehyde solution and then incubated with PV or normal IgG, followed by FITC-conjugated anti-human IgG. Right panels represent magnifications of the highlighted box within left panels. (b) Pre-incubation of PV serum with purified keratinocyte 130 kDa protein(s) abolished the staining of PV IgG on PBMC surface (left panel), whereas pre-incubation with gel pure 130 kDa protein(s) from PBMC extracts apparently did not impair keratinocyte staining by PV IgG.

To definitively exclude that this 130 kDa band corresponded to Dsg3, immunoprecipitates were assayed for Dsg3 reactivity. Western blot of the immunocomplexes using H-145 polyclonal IgG as primary antibody revealed that the 130 kDa antigen was not Dsg3 (Figure 2(e)). This finding was further ascertained by probing filters with the 5H10 and 5G11 monoclonal antibodies raised against the extracellular domain of human Dsg3 (not shown). Taken together, these findings demonstrate that PV IgG recognize an antigen synthesized by PBMC other than Dsg3 (PVA2) with molecular weight of 130 kDa.

The Novel 130 kDa Antigen Is Expressed on PBMC Surface

Immunofluorescence microscopy on permeabilized PBMC was performed in order to assess the cellular localization of PVA2. PV, BP and normal sera were incubated with PBMC and then bound antibodies were left to react with FITC-conjugated anti-human IgG. Immunofluorescence analysis revealed that PV IgG, but not Nh IgG, recognized antigen(s) located on PBMC surface (Figure 3. (a)). Indeed, FITC fluorescence appeared localized all around cell membrane, describing a fishnet-like pattern on aggregated PBMC similar to that observed in the epidermis. Moreover, when IgG from another immune-mediated bullous disease such as BP were probed as a further control, the immunostaining on PBMC was found negative (not shown), confirming that the above fluorescence features were PV-specific.

Interestingly, pre-incubation of PV IgG with gel pure 130 kDa protein(s) of keratinocyte origin abolished the PBMC fluorescence (Figure 3. (b), *PBMC*), indicating that the novel autoantigen was expressed in both keratinocytes and PBMC. It is a formal possibility that PV IgG exhibit cross-reaction between Dsg3 and PV130. On the contrary, pre-incubation with PBMC extracts did not grossly affect the reactivity of PV IgG against keratinocyte surface antigens (Figure 3. (b), *keratinocytes*). Overall, these data definitively demonstrated that PV patients can develop autoimmunity against blood cells antigen(s).

PV IgG-depleted Sera Induce Dramatic Morphological Changes on Keratinocytes

To study the effect of the non-immunoglobulin serum factors on keratinocyte morphology, we incubated cells with 50% (v/v) IgG-depleted sera. Along a 48-hours time period, keratinocytes incubated with IgG-free control serum did not show any relevant alteration of cell periphery and morphology, as revealed by FITC-staining of Dsg3 (Figure 4. (a), compare with Figure 1. (c)).

Conversely, signs of cell-cell detachment became appreciable within 24 h after treatment with IgG-free PV sera (Figure 4.(b)). Incipient cell shrinkage or obvious signs of disruption of intercellular contact were observed 48h after exposure to serum (Figure 4. (c)).

In some areas, the punctuate staining of FITC-fluorescence on cell surface, referred to as contact areas among keratinocytes, were no more detectable.

Abrogation of Dsg3 extracellular domain from membrane punctuate clusters accompanied the appearance of prickle-like processes which brought together shrinking cells (Figure 4. (c)), *arrowheads*), as shown by FITC-fluorescence.

Overall, no marked changes of nuclear morphology were found to parallel with these profound modifications of cell shape (Figure 4. (d-f). Taken together, these data demonstrate that PV sera depleted of IgG can exert remarkable effects on keratinocyte morphology.

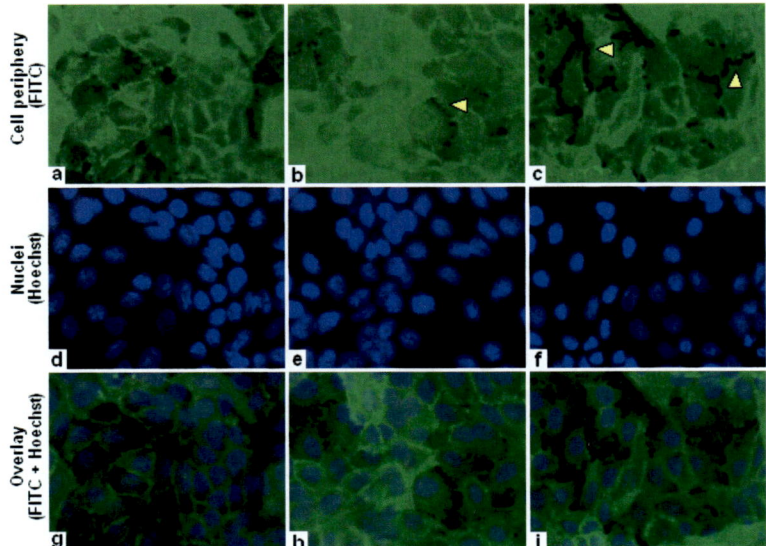

Figure 4. Effects of IgG-free sera on keratinocyte morphology. Confluent keratinocytes were incubated with IgG-depleted normal or PV sera for 24 and 48 hours and then subjected to living cell immunofluorescence microscopy, as detailed in materials and methods. Cells were stained with anti-Dsg3 antibody (cell periphery) and Hoechst (nuclei). Whole control sera depleted of IgG did not exert relevant effect on cell shape and Dsg3 distribution 48 h after treatment (a). Conversely, PV IgG-free sera affected keratinocyte morphology and cell-cell contacts within 24 h (b). Disruption of intercellular contacts, changes in Dsg3 distribution and incipient signs of cell shrinkage became evident within 48 after treatment (c, arrowheads). Overall, nuclear morphology did not appear altered (d-f).

Effects of IgG-free PV Sera on Keratinocyte Viability and Cell-Cell Adhesion

To evaluate whether serum factors other than IgG can affect metabolic activity of keratinocytes, we carried out the MTT assay on cells exposed to the sera. Cells exposed to both whole and IgG-free normal sera exhibited MTT scores comparable with controls (Figure 5).

Conversely, PV sera appeared to greatly affect keratinocyte viability. Indeed, metabolic activity decreased to about 50% of the control values (after normalization of the scores with the percentage of cell death) in keratinocytes treated with PV IgG-free sera (Figure 5).

Similar results were obtained by using whole PV sera ($p<0.05$ vs control). PV sera are thought to weak intercellular adhesion through the direct action of PV IgG, which interfere with the establishment of stabile interactions among Dsg (Mahoney et al., 1999).

To assess whether non-IgG factors in PV sera exist that affect cell-cell adhesion, a dispase-based assay was carried out. As dispase disrupts cell-matrix interactions without affecting cell-cell adhesion, incubation with 2ml dispase (0,25 %) enabled us to release keratinocytes from the substrate as a uniform monolayer. Than, cell sheets were gently placed in 15 ml conical tubes containing 2ml PBS. Tubes were rotated 30 times to expose the cell sheet to mechanical stress and then monolayer fragments were counted. Keratinocytes incubated with normal whole (n=3) and IgG-depleted (n=3) sera exhibited only minimal dissociation, whereas cells exposed to PV (n=3) sera dispersed into numerous fragments (Figure 6). The effects of IgG-free PV sera on cell adhesion were intermediate, showing dissociation rates higher than control groups but not statistically significant ($p>0.05$ versus control serum).

By and large, these results indicate that PV-specific serum factors other than autoantibodies are able to affect metabolic activity of keratinocytes and, at least partially, cell-cell adhesion.

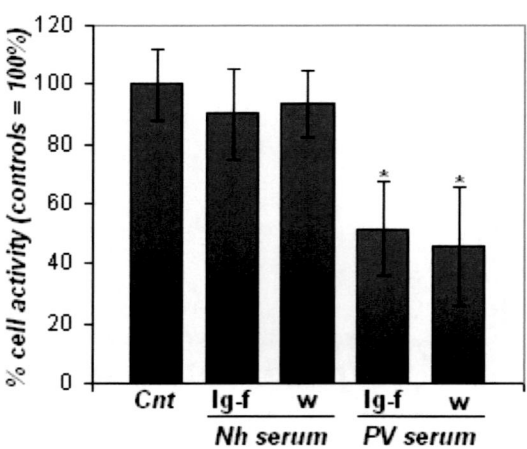

Figure 5. Metabolic assay on HaCaT cells in the presence of PV or normal sera. Cells treated with either whole or IgG-free PV sera for 36 h showed lower percentage of cell viability if compared with controls. Each experiment was performed in triplicate and the main values ± SD were represented by histograms. The average absorbance of controls was referred to as 100% cell viability. *$p<0.01$ versus control; w, whole; Ig-f, immunoglobulin-free, Nh, normal human.

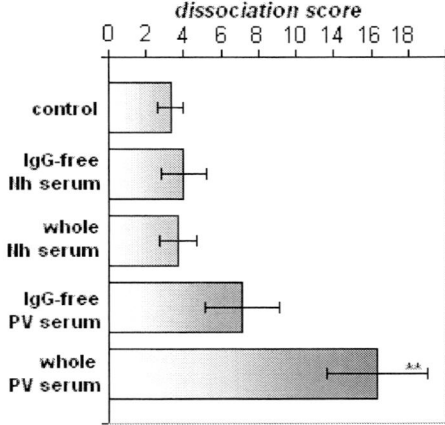

Figure 6. Effects of sera on cell-cell adhesion strength. The degree of fragmentation (dissociation score) of cell sheets was estimated by counting particles of more than 3mm. As revealed by dissociation scores, both whole and IgG-depleted PV sera weaken the intercellular adhesion strength among keratinocytes. Normal sera displayed scores comparable with control. Values are the mean of at least two independent experiments ± SD, **p<0.01.

PERK expression is altered in pemphigus vulgaris and is dependent on non-IgG factors

In keratinocytes exposed to PV sera, PERK protein levels were upregulated (P > 0.05) after 30 s (Fig. 7a, b); the peak of expression was reached within 30 s of PV serum exposure and thereafter PERK expression decreased. This correlated with transient phosphorylation of PERK, which peaked at 30 s (P < 0.05) and was virtually undetectable after 3 min (Fig. 7c). Minor levels of PERK expression and phosphorylation were also observed in keratinocytes incubated with the two control sera.

To evaluate whether the major changes in PERK levels were related to PERK activity, we examined the phosphorylation status of eIF2a, a downstream target of PERK (Fig. 7a, c). While the overall expression level of eIF2a and its phosphorylated form showed slight changes in experimental PV (n = 2) compared with controls (n = 2) after 30 s exposure to sera (P > 0.05) (Fig. 7a), eIF2a was phosphorylated (P < 0.05) 3 min after incubation with PV but not with control sera (Fig. 7c, d). Taken together, the results suggest that PERK activity is altered in experimental PV.

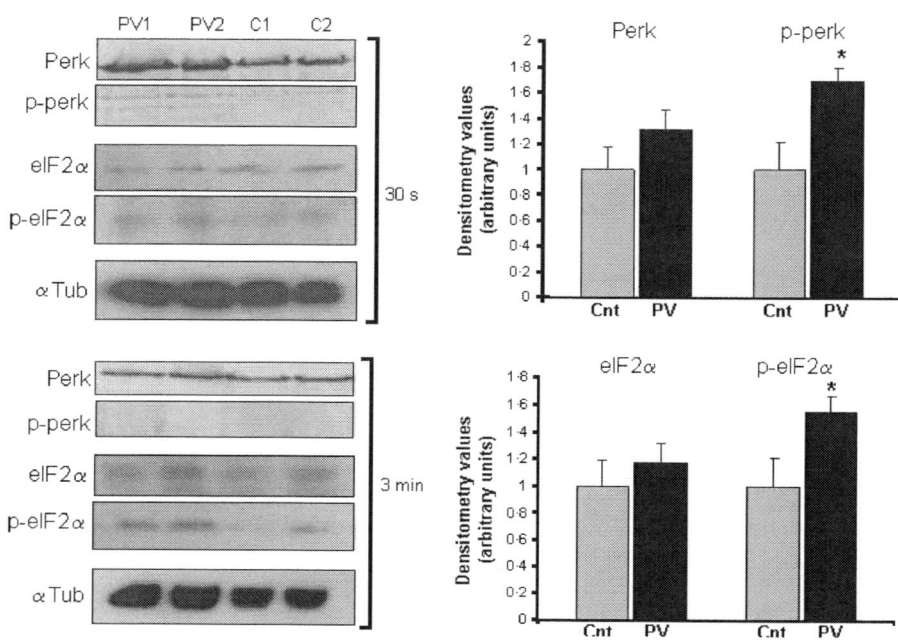

Figure 7. Western blot analysis of cell lysates from keratinocytes exposed to pemphigus vulgaris (PV) serum for 30 s and 3 min. HaCaT cells were treated with sera from individuals with PV (PV1 and PV2) or healthy controls (C1 and C2). PERK, eIF2a and their phosphorylated counterparts were investigated; α-tubulin (Tub) protein was used as a loading control. Images (a) and (c) represent the typical appearance of blots obtained in three independent experiments. Densitometric analysis was undertaken and the results from C1–2 and PV1–2 were averaged; significant results are reported as mean ± SD in (b) (30 s) and (d) (3 min). *$P < 0.05$, Cnt, control sera.

By In-Cell western blot [160], we then showed that both PERK and its phosphorylated counterpart peaked at 1 min after treatment with whole PV and PV immunoglobulin-free sera, but not PV IgG and controls; PERK and p-PERK returned to control levels within 30 min of treatment (Fig. 8). These data demonstrate that the early phosphorylation of PERK in experimental PV is attributable to non-immunoglobulin factors.

Further, cell viability and metabolic activity of keratinocytes were reduced significantly by treatment with PV immunoglobulin- free sera, but metabolic activity was restored in PERK-deficient cells (Fig. 9a, b). Cell adhesion strength was also affected by PV immunoglobulin-free sera, as demonstrated by the increase in large epithelial fragments with the dispase-based dissociation assay. Notably, treatment with PERK siRNAs reduced the number of large epithelial fragments produced by incubation with PV immunoglobulin-free sera (Fig. 9c).

Collectively, these findings provide evidence that PV sera depleted of immunoglobulins determine metabolic and functional changes in keratinocytes via mechanisms that involve PERK.

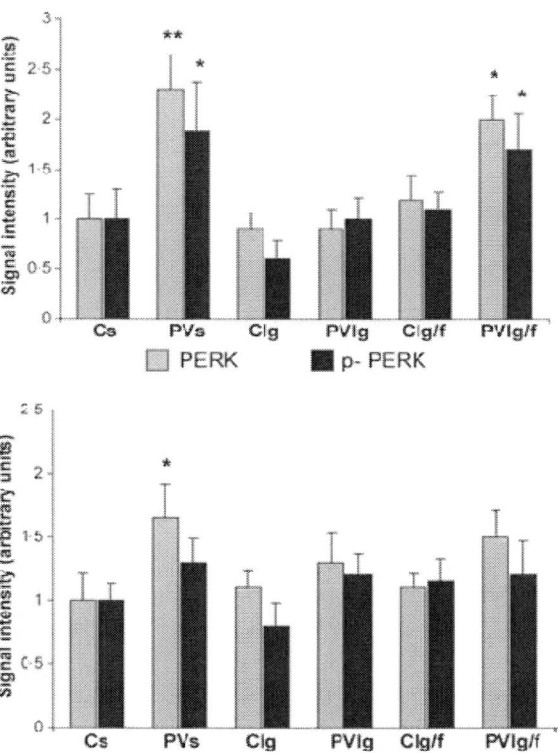

Figure 8. Expression of PERK and phosphorylated-PERK (p-PERK) by incell enzyme-linked immunosorbent assay after treatment with control sera (Cs), pemphigus vulgaris (PV) sera (PVs), control immunoglobulin (CIg), PV IgG (PVIg), control immunoglobulin-free sera (CIg /f) and PV immunoglobulin-free sera (PVIg / f) for 1 min (a) or 30 min (b). Final values were the mean of three experiments for each serum and were obtained by normalizing the fluorescence intensity for each well with the number of cells. Values for the untreated cells were arbitrarily fixed as 1. Results are shown as mean ± SD. *$P < 0.05$, **$P < 0.01$.

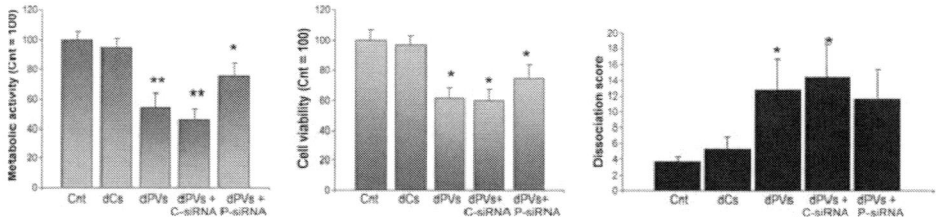

Figure 9. Cell metabolic activity (a, MTT assay), cell viability (b, trypan blue exclusion) and cell–cell adhesion (c, dispase assay) in HaCaT keratinocytes after treatment with pemphigus vulgaris immunoglobulin-free sera (PVs) in the presence (C-siRNA) or absence of PERK (P-siRNA). Controls included untreated keratinocytes (Cnt) and keratinocytes treated with control sera (Cs). Results are shown as mean ± SD. *P < 0.05, **P < 0.01.

Discussion

Recent advances in the pathophysiology of PV have unambiguously demonstrated that antidesmoglein autoimmunity acts in concert with other pathomechanisms leading to loss of cell-cell adhesion [8, 128]. This study provides the first strong evidence that *a)* blood cells can be targeted by PV autoimmunity, and *b)* non-IgG serum factors play a relevant role in the immunopathogenesis of PV.

Indeed, the results of the study of non-Dsg antigens clearly showed that PV IgG recognized a 130 kDa autoantigen other than Dsg3 located on the surface of PBMC. This novel autoantigen, PV130, seemed to be expressed also by keratinocytes, since pre-absorption with HaCat extracts strongly impaired the reactivity of PV IgG against PBMC surface. The section dealing with the role non-IgG factors in PV represents an absolute breacktrouth in the knowledge of pemphigus pathophysiology. The results of this study were obtained *in vitro* by using several experimental approaches, including (a) morphologic (b) metabolic and (c) functional analyses on keratinocytes exposed to PV sera depleted of IgG. Thus, we have successfully demonstrated that IgG-free PV sera can (a) induce dramatic changes on cell shape and drastically reduce the contact areas among keratinocytes, with the subsequent formation of appreciable gaps between contiguous cells; (b) reduce cell viability; (c) affect keratinocyte intercellular adhesion.

Under certain aspects, pemphigus represents an enigma for investigators. Although a series of paper shed light on the pathophysiological mechanisms of epithelial acantholysis [20, 67], the current explanation for pemphigus autoimmunity appears to be not completely satisfactory [118, 129]. Until the antigenic targets and their functions will not be fully elucidated, we will be unable to clarify the complex phenomena that drive the disease. Observations reported in the present paper open new roads towards a better understanding of PV autoimmunity by shifting the search from the epidermis to the blood cells. For example, the regulation of the autoimmune response by a PV antigen on PBMC could explain the inconsistency, not seldom observed, between immunological findings and clinical phenomenology.

Previous reports told about autoantigens other than Dsg1 and Dsg3 in PV [23]. Indeed, epidermis of Dsg3-null mice was found to describe a fishnet-like pattern when incubated with Dsg1-depleted PV sera on immunofluorescence analysis. The novelty of our findings consists in that the 130 kDa antigen recognized by PV IgG is located on PBMC. Hence, PV autoimmunity target non-epithelial cells which do not assemble desmosomes nor express desmogleins. Further studies will elucidate the nature of this novel 130 kDa antigen, allowing to clarify whether PV130 plays a pathogenic role in the pathophysiology of PV. However, to generalize our observations, a largest number of patients is needed.

The data from the experiments with IgG-free sera are revolutionary in that they definitively breaks the belief that IgG are the sole mediators of pemphigus and open new perspectives towards a better knowledge of the disease. In fact, our observations suggest that the pathogenesis of PV relies on complex mechanisms of action including the activity of serum factors other than IgG. In this context, our previous results suggesting that serum proteinases can be involved in enhancing tissue proteinase activity are relevant [110], although their precise contribution to the acantholysis still remains to be elucidated. So far, the autoantibody-mediated effects of PV sera have been the best studied and seemed to account for almost all PV phenomenology. However, many aspects among those claimed to demonstrate the exclusive role of IgG in PV pathogenesis are still unclear. A key element of dogma on the exclusive role of IgG in PV blister formation is represented by the transitory, self-limited blister eruption observed in neonates born by mothers with active pemphigus [130]. However, our investigations have established that low molecular mass (<50 kDa) factors present in the sera of PV patients can induce on their own specific changes on keratinocytes. Consistently, one can speculate that acantholytic serum factors of <50 kDa in size may penetrate the placenta and contribute to the pathogenesis of neonatal pemphigus. Other incongruence of the current theories also depends upon the fact that, although

PV antigens are present throughout the epidermis, yet blister formation occurs in definite areas. This suggests the intervention of local factors in the pathophysiology of acantholysis. Keratinocyte-derived cytokines might be this lacking plug, being induced and/or cooperating with serum cytokines in creating a microenvironment permissive for acantholysis. Further studies will address whether these serum factors are "permissive", "precipitating", or "pathogenic" for PV acantholysis. The present scenario also arises important methodological issues. In fact, he experimental models used to reproduce the disease seems questionable. The amount of purified PV IgG usually chosen for *in vivo* experiments is very high, corresponding to a concentration 10-20-fold greater than that of physiologically occurring serum gamma globulins [108]. On the other hand, the use of anti-Dsg3 IgG would appear inadequate, as revealed by the lack of spontaneous blistering in the mouse model injected with anti-Dsg3 antibody alone as well as the finding that mice immunized with full-length Dsg3 did not develop lesions [107]. In light of our data, the use of whole sera for reproducing the experimental models of PV seems to be warranted.

In summary, here we provided the first evidence that PV IgG recognize antigen(s) located outside the epidermis. The novel PV autoantigen, PV130, is found on both PBMC surface and keratinocytes but, although displaying a molecular mass of 130 kDa, it is not Dsg3. Furthermore, we established for the first time well-defined changes caused by PV IgG-free sera on keratinocytes. Indeed, PV sera depleted of IgG were able to induce distinct and reproducible morphological, metabolic and functional alterations *in vitro*. Thus, we concluded that PV-specific phenomena such as cell shrinkage, disruption of cell-cell contacts, and reduction of cell viability relies on the cooperating action of both PV IgG and serum factors other than IgG. These data have remarkable consequences on both experimental models of PV and its therapy, as now it has become clear that PV acantholysis is not the result of the exclusive activity of IgG: PV pathophysiology cannot be faithfully reproduced by leaving serum factors out of consideration.

Chapter 6

Downstream Signaling Involved in Acantholysis: Part I: Changes in Cell Cycle and Protein Phosphorylation

Autoantibodies present in PV patients can promote detrimental effects by triggering altered transduction of signals which results in a final acantholysis. Over the last few years it has been demonstrated that enhanced kinase activity appears to be involved in cytoskeleton organization and cell adhesion.

Furthermore, phosphorylation of desmosomal proteins is known to regulate the dynamic of desmosome assembly/disassembly to the sites of intercellular contact To investigate mechanisms involved in PV, cultured keratinocytes were treated with PV serum.

By using a phosphoprotein assay kit, here we show that PV serum affects cell phosphorylation status. In particular, we individuated three specific phosphorylation events.

Furthermore, PV sera were able to promote the cell cycle progression inducing the accumulation of cyclin-dependent kinase 2 (cdk2). This overexpression was shown both *in vitro* by Western blotting and *in vivo* on patients' skin.

Interestingly, small interfering RNA depletion of cdk2 prevented disruption of cell-cell adhesion. Thus, a new pathogenic scenario for CDK2-dependent alterations in acantholysis present PV and other diseases should be investigated

Introduction

Despite years of research on PV pathophysiology, to date precise molecular mechanisms underlying acantholysis have not yet been fully understood.

Until recently, it was believed that disruption of cell-cell contacts resulted from the simple interaction of PV autoantibodies with Dsgs by steric hindrance [2].

However, today this model appear untenable, as: a) autoimmunity in PV is not just restricted to adhesion molecules [8], b) serum factors other than IgG could play a role in PV pathogenesis [127] and c) a number of signal-transduction cascades seem to be crucially involved in acantholysis [87-89]. With regard to this, an emerging concept is that phosphorylation events could be impaired in PV.

Consistently, activation of signalling through both protein kinase C (PKC) isoforms and p38 mitogen activated protein kinase (MAPK) have been proposed to initiate acantholytic changes by inducing desmosome disassembling and cytoskeleton reorganization [37, 87]. Protein phosphorylation is one of the most rapid post-translational modifications engaged by the cell in order to modulate protein activity, localization, and stability.

Over the last few years it has been demonstrated that enhanced kinase activity appears to be involved in cytoskeleton organization and cell adhesion [37, 38]. Furthermore, phosphorylation of desmosomal proteins is known to regulate the dynamic of desmosome assembly/disassembly to the sites of intercellular contact [14].

Phosphorylation events are controlled by protein kinases, which can regulate the onset and transition through mitosis [131]. Thus, PV sera may influence the cell-cycle progression of keratinocytes.

One of the central kinases involved in G1 regulation is the cyclin-dependent kinase 2 (cdk2), an essential component of the cell cycle machine, which can be altered in several diseases, such as cancer, and gestational trophoblastic disease [132-134].

To date, no precise correlations between PV and keratinocyte cell-cycle progression have been established. The goal of the present study was to investigate the pathogenic molecular events involved in PV.

Materials and Methods

Antibodies and Reagents

Polyclonal IgG against perk, p-perk, Akt, p-Akt, Ask1, αPAK, p-αPAK, jak1, cdk2, PKR, p-PKR, p-p38, CK1, Dsg1, STE-20, β-actin, pancytokeratin, and horse radish peroxidase (HRP)-conjugated anti-rabbit and anti-mouse IgG were from Santa Cruz Biotecnology (Santa Cruz, CA). Nitrocellulose membranes were purchased from Invitrogen (Carlsbad, CA); reagents for enhanced chemiluminescence (ECL) and films were from Amersham (Buckinghamshire, U.K.). All reagents used for protein extraction and cell cultures were obtained from Sigma (St. Louis, MO), except keratinocyte growth medium (KGM) and antibiotics/antimicotic, purchased from Gibco BRL (Gaithersburg, MD).

Keratinocyte Culture Experiments

On the basis of both our preliminary experiments with PV IgG and other studies [42], we preferred to set experiments in the presence of PV serum instead of isolated IgG. Primary human keratinocytes were isolated from tongue specimens of patients undergoing glossoplasty, as detailed in chapter 2. Primary keratinocytes and HaCaT were growth at 37°C in an atmosphere humidified with 5% CO_2. At the time of the experiment, cells were seeded on 35mm Petri plastic dishes and growth to confluence.

The standard protocols for treatment of keratinocyte monolayers with pemphigus serum were followed (chapter 2). For reproducing the *in vitro* model of PV on cellcultures, keratinocytes were incubated with 30% sera from PV patients and controls for 24, 48 or 72 hours.

Cell Cycle Analysis

In order to study major effects of PV serum on keratinocyte cell cycle, we have synchronized HaCat keratinocytes with 0,5% of FBS for 24 hours. The starvation method has been set by the use of a colorimetric immunoassay based on the measurement of BrdU incorporation during DNA synthesis (Cell proliferation ELISA, Roche). Synchronized and unsynchronized cells have been treated with PV serum (30%) and normal serum (30%) for 24 hours.

Fresh cells were pretreated with 100 g/ml RNAase for 30 min at 37°C and stained with 20 g/ml propidium iodide before flow cytometric analysis (FACSCalibur; Becton Dickinson, Milan, Italy).

Western Blot Analysis

Fifty µg cytosolic extracts of sample were separated by 8-12% sodium dodecyl sulphate (SDS)-polyacrylamide gel electrophoresis (PAGE) and transferred to nitrocellulose membranes as described (25-27). Western blotting and immunoprecipitation were performed as detailed by us elsewhere (chapter 2).

Protein Phosphorylation Assay

For phosphoprotein assay, proteins extracted with Triton buffer (20mM Tris-HCl, pH 7.5, 150 mM NaCl, 5 mM EDTA, 1% Triton X-100, 1 mM DTT, 1 mM PMSF, 10 µg/ml leupeptin and 10 µg/ml aprotinin) were delipidated and desalted as follows: 600 µl methanol, 150 µl chloroform 450 µl deionised water were added to 150 µl cell lysates adjusted to contain equal amount of protein and vortexed. Mixture was centrifuged at 16,000 x g for 5 min, then the supernatant was discarded and pellets left to dry on open air before resuspending them in 1X Laemmli sample buffer. Proteins (250 µg per lane) were resolved by 10% SDS-PAGE and transferred on nitrocellulose membranes. Filters were fixed in 7% acetic acid/ 10% methanol (v/v) and subsequently stained with the phosphoprotein stain solution, according to the manufacturer's instructions. Bands on dried filters were visualized using UV illumination and signal intensities quantified by Molecular Analysis Software (*Bio-Rad*).

siRNA Treatment

CDK2-directed siRNA pool (L-003236) and negative control pool (D-001206-13-05) were purchased from Dharmacon, Inc. (Lafayette, CO). The siRNAs were transfected at final concentration of 100 nM using Dharmafect 1 according to the manufacturer's recommendations. The siRNAs were incubated with glass-coverslips cultured HaCaT cells over night. Afterwards, cells were treated with 30% PV and 30% control sera for both 24 and 48 hours and then formalin fixed for immunofluorescence studies. The efficiency of transfection was monitored by using siglo cyclophilin B as control (D-001610-01-05) as well as by Western blot for CDK2 expression.

Immunofluorescence and Immunohistochemistry

Immunofluorescence studies were carried out as described previously (chapter 3). Formalin fixed, paraffine embedded skin biopsies from pemphigus patients were subjected to immunohistochemical analysis as described in detail [104].

Morphometric Analysis of Cell-Cell Detachment

The extent of cell detachment (acantholysis) in cell monolayers was measured by modifying previously published protocols, as reported in chapter 2.

Results

PV Sera Affect Cell Phosphorylation Status

Changes in protein phosphorylation state may be the physiological expression of cell cycle progression. Hence, to exclude that results were biased by disomogeneous cell cycle-related events, we carried out the set of inhibitor experiments on synchronized cells enriched in S phase (see materials and methods). Keratinocytes were incubated in pilot assays with 30% or 50% (v/v) PV or normal sera for 1, 30 min, 3, 6, 24 and 48 h. After determining optimal conditions, phosphoproteins from cell lysates were analyzed at 1 min, 3- and 24-hour time points by using the Pro-Q® Diamond Phosphoprotein Kit. This assay provides a simple method for directly detecting phosphoproteins on nitrocellulose membranes. Results showed that PV serum was specifically responsible for transient changes in the protein phosphorilation pattern of keratinocytes (Figure 1. and Figure 2). Two proteins of apparent molecular masses of ~35 and ~45 kDa were found to be transiently phosphorylated within 1 min after exposure to 50% PV serum (Figure 1. (a) *PV serum*). A strong phosphorylation event occurred within 3 hours of incubation with PV serum and seemed to involve a ~80 kDa protein (Figure 1. (a)). Densitometry values are provided in Figure 2. (*PVs*). However, cell phosphorylation state did not show any significant change in comparison with controls 24 hours after serum treatment (Figure 1. (a)). None of the observed phosphorylation patterns paralleled with changes in keratinocyte morphology, as revealed by immunofluorescence microscopy. In fact, while kinase machinery seemed to be activated within 1 min after exposure to PV serum, no alterations of cell shape were detected by immunofluorescence within 6 hours of treatment (Figure 1. (b)). Keratinocytes started to shrink after 24 hours, and were grossly detached from one another within 48 hours after PV sera exposure. Typical acantholytic dismorphisms included rounding up, keratinocyte-keratinocyte detachment and dramatic Dsg3 redistribution. FITC staining was strongly revealed along the otherwise intact nuclear periphery, whereas it was depleted from cell surface (Figure 1. (a)). Impact of normal serum on changes in protein phosphorilation state (Figure 1. (a) *normal serum*) and cell morphology (Figure 1. (b)) was weak. The three specific events induced by PV serum were decreases or abrogated in the presence of 100nM STS, a broad kinase inhibitor (Figure 2). Taken together, these data demonstrate that PV sera induce specific phosphorylation events in keratinocytes.

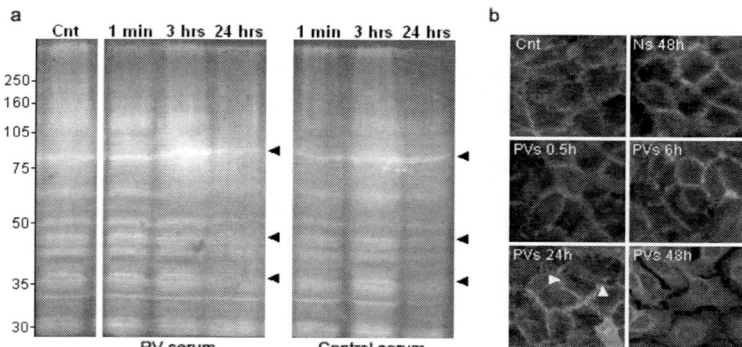

Figure 1. As (a) Keratinocytes were incubated with PV or normal sera for 1 min, 3 hrs or 24 hrs and then harvested and subjected to protein extraction and phosphoprotein assay. (b) For immunofluorescence studies, cells were exposed to sera for 30 min, 6 hrs, 24 hrs, and 48 hrs. PV serum, but not control serum, was able to induce keratinocyte acantholysis. However, first signs of disruption of cell-cell contacts were observed after 24 hours, whereas gross changes such as rounding up of keratinocytes, and redistribution of Dsg3 staining, became obvious after 48 hours. Figure was representative of independent experiments carried out by probing all sera.

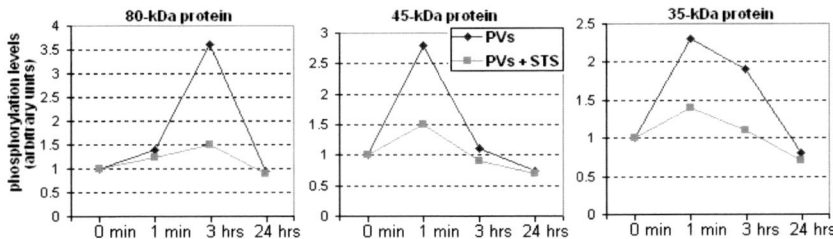

Figure 2. Cells were cultured with PV serum for the indicated time points with or without staurosporine (STS). Figure shows densitometry values against the three PV-specific phosphorilation events. It represents the mean value of three independent experiments.

PV serum promotes activation of a number protein kinases in keratinocytes

The expression of selected kinases belonging to different branches of kinome was evaluated by Western blots. We determined optimal conditions in pilot assays and then incubated cells for 1, 3, 10, 30, 60, and 180 min with PV or control sera (then the supplemented medium was removed and replaced with normal medium). Within 1 min after exposure to serum, perk was found to be upregulated by PV sera (called PV1-PV4) (Figure 3. (a)).

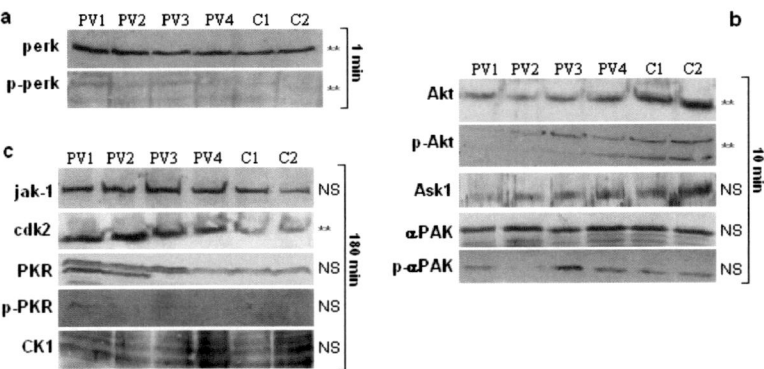

Figure 3. Sera of PV patients induce changes in kinase expression. Western blot of keratinocyte lysates at 1, 10, and 180 min after incubation with 30% PV or control sera (a-c). Significant changes in perk (1 min) Akt, p-Akt (10 min), cdk2, and jak-1 expression were revealed. Figures were representative of three independent

experiments. P, patients; C, healthy controls; *, p<0.05; **, p<0.01; NS, non significant.

On the other hand, Akt and Ask1 levels diminished in PV-treated cells in comparison with controls within 10 min (Figure 3. (b)). Phosphorylation of Akt was virtually abolished in cells exposed to PV sera. Later events included jak-1, cdk2 and PKR overexpression (Figure 3. (c)). On the basis of these preliminary findings, we chose to investigate more in depth those kinases showing higher responsivity to PV serum. Cumulative densitometric analysis revealed a significant increase of perk expression (and its phosphorylated form) after exposure to PV sera, although this phenomenon was variable (for example exposure to PV3 serum induced modest effects). This phenomenon was more evident in another independent experiment showed in Figure 4. (a) in which both expression and phosphorylation of perk reached the peak within 30 sec after transient exposure to PV sera, whereas their level became virtually indistinguishable from controls in 3-min treated cells.

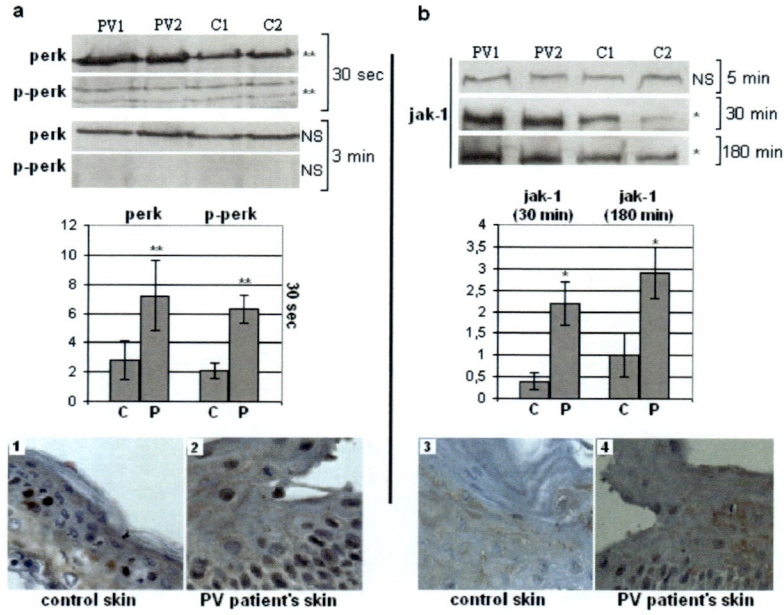

Figure 4. Time course studies revealed a significant but transient phosphorylation of perk together with its overexpression (a). Jak-1 protein levels were also transiently increased (b). Densitometry values (histograms) were obtained by using β-actin protein levels (=10) as a control. Figures were representative of three independent experiments. P, patients; C, healthy controls; *p<0.05; **p<0.01; NS, not significant.

Consistently, immunohistochemistry analysis on skin biopsies from patients with PV (n=3) showed diffuse upregulation of perk in lesional and perilesional epidermis (2) in comparison with healthy skin (1).

Perk expression was then investigated by immunohistochemistry on skin biopsies from patients with PV (n=3). Analysis of immunostaining showed diffuse upregulation of perk in lesional and perilesional epidermis in PV patients (Figure 4. (a-1)(a-2)). Jak-1 exhibited a slow increase, showing a progressive upregulation along the 180 min incubation with PV sera (Figure 4. (b)). Expression of jak-1 protein was further investigated by immunohistochemistry on skin biopsies from patients with PV. jak-1 immunostaining was restricted to the perilesional areas of patient's skin, but not around the acantholytic cleft (Figure 4. (b-3) (b-4)).

Cell Cycle Analysis

Among the array of protein kinases subjected to screening, we found a marked up-regulation of cell-cycle-related kinases, including cdk2. Thus, to analyze major effects of PV serum on cell-cycle progression in keratinocytes, we have treated synchronized cells with PV serum (30%) for 24 hours (Figure 5 a, b). Interestingly, PV-treated samples displayed a lower percentage of cells in G1 phase in comparison with controls. Concomitantly, the number of cells in S phase were significantly higher after treatment with PV serum if compared with normal serum. Also, experiments revealed a lower percentage of cells in G2 phase, indicating a selective increase of cell cycle progression. Thus, PV serum enhances the G1/S transition with subsequent accumulation of cells in S phase.

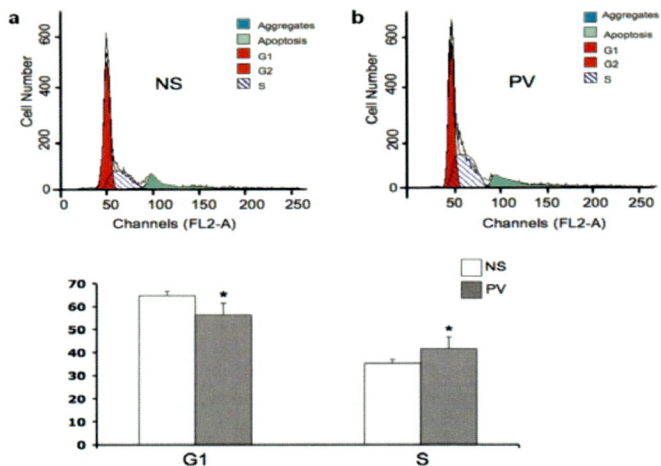

Figure 5. (previous page). Cell cycle analysis of cultured keratinocytes treated with normal (a) or PV (b) sera. Synchronic HaCaT keratinocytes treated with PV serum showed a faster progression through the cell cycle in comparison with same cells treated with normal serum (NS).

PV Sera Modulate Dose-Dependently cdk2 Expression but Modestly Other Kinases

Western blot revealed that PV serum induced a strong 10-fold increase of cdk2 expression in keratinocytes compared with normal serum (Figure 6a, b).

To further investigate correlations between PV serum (10% and 30%) and cdk2 levels, we carried out extensive experiments by incubating cells with PV and normal sera at selected time points. Keratinocytes exposed to lower quantities (10% v/v) of PV sera exhibited a less sustained up-regulation of cdk2 levels in comparison with those incubated with higher concentrations (30%) of PV serum (Figure 6c). In both conditions (10% and 30%), PV sera strongly increased the amount of cdk2 if compared with control sera, as revealed by densitometry analysis (Figure 6c).

Pilot experiments conducted with PV isolated IgG (instead of serum) showed a similar pattern of cdk2 overexpression (data not shown). To evaluate whether major changes in cdk2 levels seen in cultured cells were also appreciable *in vivo*, we performed immunohistochemical investigations on skin biopsies from PV patients and healthy controls. Data (n=4 of PV patients and healthy subjects, n=2) confirmed the assumption that cdk2 was overexpressed in skin of PV patients (Figure 6d). A positive staining on the basal cell layer was not unexpected, since basal keratinocytes are active mitotically (Figure 6 (d-1)). PV patient skin showed an intense staining just around the site of the acantholytic cleft (Figure 6 (d-3, d-4)). Furthermore, there was an increase of cdk2 expression along suprabasal layers in perilesional sites (unaffected skin) (Figure 6 (d-2)) indicating that cdk2 up-regulation may precede blister formation.

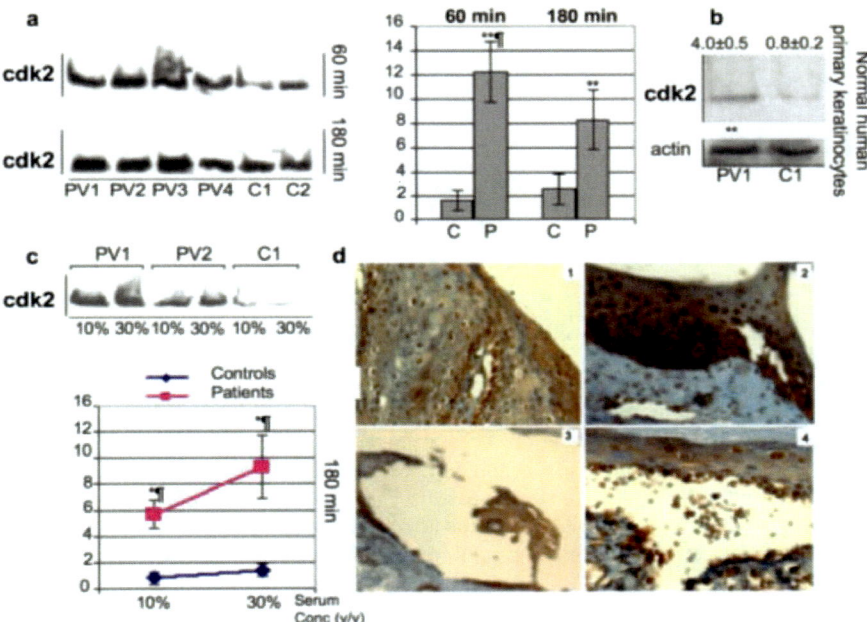

Figure 6. Significant increase in CDK2 expression in both HaCaT keratinocytes (a) and primary normal human keratinocytes (b), as revealed by Western blotting. CDK2 overexpression was demonstrated to be a dose-dependent phenomenon, as shown by incubation of HaCaT cells with either 10% or 30% sera for 180 min (c). Immunohistochemical analysis displayed intense staining in PV skin (d-2) in comparison with healthy tissues (d-1). Marked CDK2 labelling was revealed throughout basal and suprabasal layers in apparently unaffected skin as well as along the floor and the periphery of the blister (d-3, 4). Densitometry values (histograms) were normalized by using β-actin protein (=10) as a control. Western blotting was representative of three independent experiments. P, patients; C, healthy controls; *, $p<0.05$; **, $p<0.01$; *, $p<0.005$; **, $p<0,001$; NS, non significant.

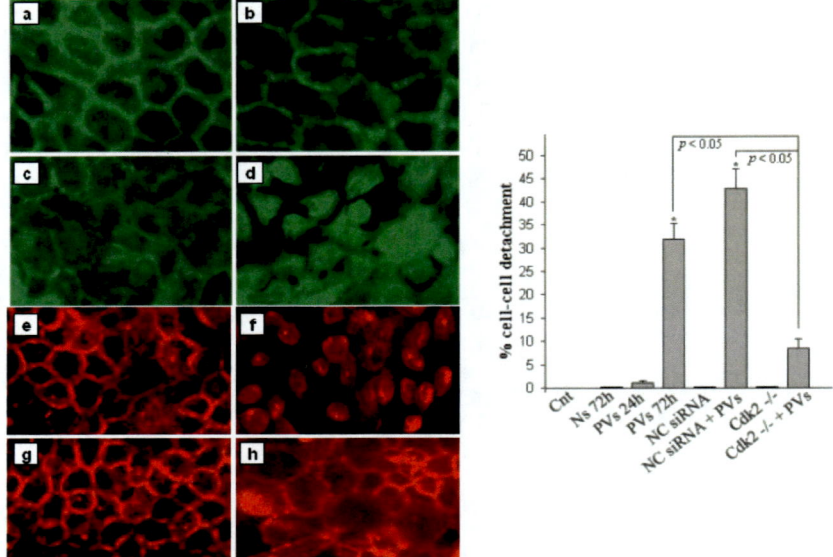

Figure 7. Lack of CDK2 prevents cell-cell detachment induced by PV sera. As revealed by immunofluorescence microscopy, cells incubated with control sera did not show any morphological alteration or rearrangement of Dsg1 within 72 hs after treatment (a,b). Conversely, first changes in cell shape became evident within 24 hs after treatment with PV sera, as revealed by formation of prickle-like processes associated with cell shrinkage (c). 72 hs after incubation with PV sera cells were clearly detached from one another and rounded up (D). Effect of CDK2-specific siRNAs on HaCaT cell-cell detachment induced by PV sera (e-h). CDK2-directed siRNA pool (G-H) and negative control siRNAs pool (e-f) were transfected and treated with PV (f-h) and control serum (e-g) for 24 hs before immunofluorescence analysis with the Dsg1 antibody. (I) Ten fields of different photograms were used to calculate the mean values of cell-cell detachment by morphometric analysis.

Silencing of cdk2 Prevents Cell-Cell Detachment Induced by PV Sera

Keratinocyte monolayers were exposed to whole PV and control sera for 24 and 72 hours, then we tested the ability of PV sera to induce cell-cell detachment. An antibody to Dsg1 was used for immunostaining of desmosomes in HaCat monolayers. Immunofluorescence performed on cultured cells revealed that incubation with 30% PV serum induced changes in cell shape within 24 h (Figure 7a, b). Punctate clusters of FITC-fluorescence on cell surface, referred to as contact areas among keratinocytes, appeared as elongated processes which brought together shrinking cells (Figure 7c).

Keratinocytes appeared completely detached from one another (Figure 7d). Some cellular processes extending from keratinocyte surface were still recognizable; however, no signs of punctuate clusters were detectable (Figure 7d). In our experimental conditions, cdk2 silencing induced a decrease of around 70% of its expression (data not shown).

To evaluate if the silencing of cdk2 prevents cell-cell detachment induced by PV sera, keratinocytes were transfected overnight with control pool siRNA and cdk2-specific siRNAs, treated for 24 hours with 30% PV serum (Figure 7f-h) and 30% control normal serum (Figure 7e-g). All the keratinocytes appeared with a normal shape when they were treated with cdk2-specific siRNA pool and negative control siRNAs pool (Figure 7g-h) in presence of control normal serum (Figure 7e-g). In the negative control, the cell detachment was more evident in comparison with cdk-specific siRNA cells. The incubation of cells with PV in cells transfected with negative control siRNAs pool induced a significant change in cell shape (Figure 7f), whereas the incubation with cdk2-specific siRNA pool promoted a partial protection from cell-cell detachment induced by PV sera (Figure 7g). Indeed, the morphometric analysis of cell-cell detachment on keratinocytes showed that the silencing of cdk2 reduced cell-cell detachment induced by PV sera to approximately 8% (Figure 7i). Data at 48 hours were not different from those of 24 hours and therefore not showed.

Discussion

The major finding of the present experimental section is that PV serum can induce specific changes in protein phosphorylation status. In particular, kinase machinery alterations occurring in PV acantholysis crucially involve cdk2. This evidence was obtained both in cultured cells and *in vivo*, by using skin biopsies of PV patients. We observed also that PV serum increased the cell cycle progression. Second, we revealed that silencing of cdk2 was able to reduce disruption of cell-cell contacts in keratinocytes exposed to PV serum.

When keratinocytes are exposed to purified PV IgG, Dsg3 is markedly phosphorylated [43]. In addition, PV IgG increase the level of phosphorylation of other adhesion molecules, such as E-cadherin, beta and gamma catenins [135]. Contextually, at least two kinase pathways become activated, whose evidence is given by the rapid and sustained increase in PKC activity and p38 MAPK phosphorilation [37, 38]. In this study, we demonstrated for the first time that PV serum can induce at least three phosphorylation events in keratinocyte proteins. These proteins showed an apparent molecular mass of ~35 kDa, ~45 kDa, and ~80 kDa. The observed changes in the cell phosphorylation status were early and transient, since two of the three proteins were phosphorylated within 1 minute of exposition to PV serum. In contrast, the first changes in cell shape were appreciated 24 hours after exposure to PV serum. Thus, changes in protein phosphorylation did not parallel with changes in cell morphology. This finding suggests that crucial molecular events, including protein phosphorylation, do occur early after exposure to serum, whereas the phenotypic results of the acantholytic cascade is a late event in PV phenomenology.

Our complete set of experiments also showed that some specific kinases may be involved in PV-induced acantholysis. Indeed, the earliest specific changes of protein phosphorylation occurred within 30 sec from exposure to PV sera. One explanation for such a rapid increase in PERK expression may be due to its enhanced phosphorylation state, with subsequent reduction of its degradation rates. Therefore, activation of perk could be one of the primary signaling pathways involved in acantholysis, although further studies are needed to address this point.

Cdk2 overexpression was demonstrated in suprabasal layers of perilesional (unaffected) skin, indicating that PV-induced changes in cdk2 levels may precede the phenotypic manifestations of disease. The sustained overexpression of cdk2 (12-fold increase) led us to investigate whether this key cell cycle regulator was causally related to PV acantholysis. Thus, we knocked-out cdk2 from keratinocytes through silencing techniques and then tested the ability of PV sera to induce adhesion loss in such a cdk2-deficient cell line. Interestingly, the absence of cdk2 conferred resistance to the action of PV serum, as keratinocytes lacking cdk2 did not develop acantholysis *in vitro*. In previous studies, Caldelari and colleagues used a similar targeted approach and reported that plakoglobin knockout keratinocytes were unresponsive to PV IgG [67]. However, they established PG $^{-/-}$ cell cultures from mouse skin. Thus, our study is the first working silencing gene approach to study the pathophysiology of PV in human keratinocytes. Here, we have exposed cultured cells to PV patient sera as proposed by Swanson and Dahl [100]. On the basis of both our preliminary experiments with PV IgG and other studies [105, 115], we preferred to avoid "nonphysiological" experimental conditions and, then, set the complete panel of experiments in the presence of PV serum instead of isolated IgG.

Results reported here revealed cdk2 to be a key protein in PV pathogenesis and opened new perspectives toward a more targeted therapy of the disease. Indeed, the current treatment of PV patients is based on the non-selective use of steroideal and immunosuppressive agents [1]. Our findings implicate that the molecular effects of PV could be targeted by using selective cdk2 inhibitors. However, safety approach of such inhibitors in humans must be properly addressed. Among novel therapeutic approaches, adjuvant B-cell depletion by rituximab is effective in otherwise therapy-resistant bullous autoimmune disorders, including PV, but may be associated with substantial adverse effects including fatal outcomes [136, 137].

Finally, it has been long believed that cdk2 binds to cyclin E or cyclin A and exclusively promotes the G1/S phase transition and that Cdc2/cyclin B complexes play a major role in mitosis. There is now evidence that Cdc2 binds to cyclin E (in addition to cyclin A and B) and is able to promote the G1/S transition (reviewed in ref. 138). This novel concept indicates that both Cdk2 and/or Cdc2 can drive cells through G1/S phase in parallel. Thus, a new pathogenic scenario for CDK2-dependent alterations in acantholysis present PV and other diseases should be investigated.

Chapter 7

Downstream Signaling Involved in Acantholysis: Part II: Secretion of Proteinases and the "Specific Proteolysis Hypothesis" of Pemphigus

Transduction of signals to the cell triggered by PV serum may induce proteinase up-regulation potentially responsible for disruption of epidermal adhesion and, ultimately, blister formation. Microarray analysis on skin from neonatal mice receiving PV serum has suggested that the equilibrium between extracellular proteinases and their inhibitors moved towards enhanced proteolytic activity in PV mouse model, at least on the transcriptional level (chapter 8). Here, we sought to investigate this hypothesis by using both *in vivo* and *in vitro* models of PV. The effects of PV serum on the protein level were studied *in vitro* both in keratinocyte monolayers and skin organ cultures focusing on matrix metalloproteinase (MMP) 9 expression and activity. By means of western blotting, zymography, and living cell immunofluorescence studies, we showed that MMP-9 was early overexpressed in keratinocytes exposed to PV serum, and subsequently secreted in the culture medium. However, we failed to demonstrate extracellular activation of MMP-9, since it was found in its 92 kDa inactive form in serum-free culture supernatants. By pharmacological approaches, we also showed that MMP-9 could actively cleave Dsg3 in apoptotic keratinocytes. Taken together, our data demonstrated that proteinase expression, particularly of MMP-9, is modulated by PV serum and associated with PV acantholysis.

Introduction

Early studies suggested that blister formation was mediated by release of non-lysosomal proteases, such as plasminogen activator (PA), secondary to antibody binding [45]. Although plasmin appeared to be the active enzyme in producing acantholysis [139], it is now accepted that neither plasmin nor plasminogen activators are necessary for pemphigus IgG-mediated acantholysis in mice [49].

Nevertheless, proteases other than plasmin could be involved in PV acantholysis. Matrix metalloproteinases (MMPs) are a family of zinc-containing endopeptidases that are either secreted or expressed at the cell surface of a number of cell types. MMPs are produced as zymogens, with a propeptide segment removed extracellularly by proteases such as plasmin, and show wide proteolytic activity and overlapping specificities. Given this complexity, it is not surprising that multiple roles for MMPs have been proposed, including regulation of cell migration, proliferation and death [140]. In particular, MMP-9 has been shown to mediate extracellular proteolysis of cell-cell contacts during apoptosis [94, 141]. In the present section, we have investigated changes of MMP-9 expression and localization in both *in vitro* and *in vivo* models of PV. MMP-9 is infact involved in the cleavage of Dsg3 during apoptosis [94]. Thus, we have studied Dsg3 in apoptotic keratinocytes to better understand the proteolytic specificity of MMP-9 against Dsg3. Apoptosis was triggered by staurosporine (STS), a chemical which showed several advantages as a programmed cell death inducer [142], including its ability to trigger apoptosis in a broad spectrum of cell types.

Materials and Methods

Keratinocyte Culture Experiments

The standard protocols for treatment of keratinocyte monolayers with pemphigus serum were followed (chapter 2). For reproducing the *in vitro* model of PV on cell cultures, keratinocytes were incubated with 30% sera from PV patients and controls for 24, 48 or 72 hours. Apoptosis was induced by addition of 800 nM staurosporine in DMSO.

Quantitation of Apoptosis

Apoptosis was assessed by nuclear morphology analysis according to the procedures reported previously [143], with some modifications. Briefly, HaCaT or HT-29 floating or adherent cells were collected 24 hours after treatment with STS and fixed in 4% formaldehyde solution for 10 min. Cells were then washed in PBS and stained with the nuclear dye DAPI (2 µg/ml) for 20 min.

Condensed/fragmented appearance of nuclear morphology (at least 100 nuclei for sample) was examined by immunofluorescence microscopy with an excitation wavelength of 355-425 nm. Apoptotic nuclei were scored based on the appearance of at least one of three different morphologies: chromatin condensation = chromatin margination without nuclear condensation; nuclear fragmentation = chromatin margination with nuclear condensation; nuclear condensation = nuclear condensation without chromatin margination. The percent cell death in each sample was calculated based on the following formula: number of apoptotic nuclei/(number of normal nuclei + number of apoptotic nuclei) x 100. Each experiment was performed in triplicate.

Western Blot Analysis and Immunofluorescence

Fifty µg cytosolic extracts of sample were separated by 8-12% sodium dodecyl sulphate (SDS)-polyacrylamide gel electrophoresis (PAGE) and transferred to nitrocellulose membranes. Western blotting, immunoprecipitation and immunofluorescence were performed as detailed in chapter 3.

Zymography

Keratinocytes were exposed for 24h to PV or normal sera. Then, serum-free conditioned medium (SFCM) was generated by incubating cells overnight in fresh serum-free DMEM. MMP-9 secretion and activity were determined in unconcentrated SFCM derived from confluent monolayers (1×10^6 cells) using

SDS-polyacrylamide gel zymography. In brief, 15 ml aliquots of SFCM were mixed with 5 ml 4x Lemmli sample buffer. After heating at 52°C for 10 min, samples were electrophoresed on a 10% SDS-polyacrylamide gel containing 0,5 mg/ml gelatin.

Once completed, gels were washed three times in 2.5% Triton X-100 for 10 min to remove SDS and then incubated overnight at 37°C in substrate buffer (50 mM Tris-HCl, pH 7.8; 10 mM $CaCl_2$, 0.1% Triton X-100). Next day, gels were washed, stained with Comassie Blue R-250 and briefly destained in 40%metanol-10% glacial acetic acid solution. Proteolytic activity appeared as clear bands on a blue background.

Results

MMP-9 Is over-Expressed in Keratinocyte Mololayers Exposed to PV Serum

MMP-9 is one of the main candidates in the acantholytic process, given its ability to cleave some extracellular components of the cell-cell adhesion structures [141]. Furthermore, the enhanced function of MMP-3 suggested by microarray data (see chapter 8) led us to further focus on MMP-9 activity, as this protease is efficiently activated just by MMP-3 in physiologic conditions.

The effects of PV serum on MMP-9 expression were first tested on HaCaT monolayers.

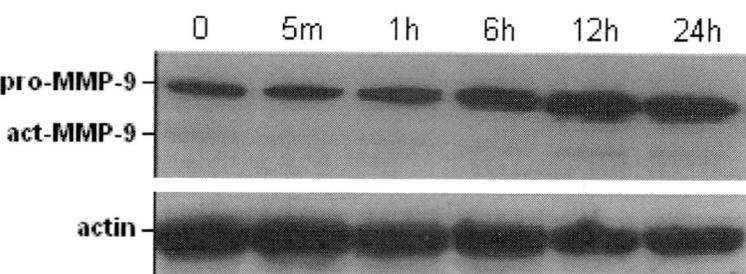

Figure 1. Sera of pemphigus vulgaris (PV) patients induce overexpression of matrix metalloproteinase 9 (MMP-9). Western blotting of HaCaT cell lysates after incubation with 30% concentrated PV sera shows a time-dependent increase of MMP-9 expression. The peak was reached 12 h after serum exposure. Western blot analysis was performed twice, giving comparable results.

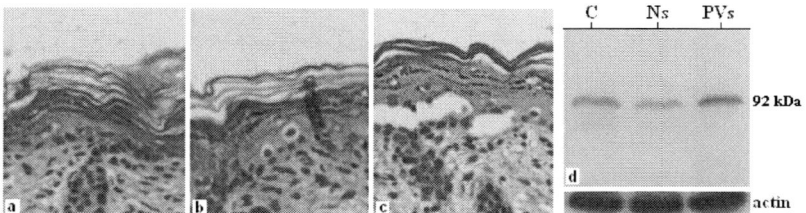

Figure 2. MMP-9 protein is up-regulated in the skin organ culture model of PV. Organ cultures were established from skin tissues of neonatal mice (a) and then exposed to PV (c) or normal (b) sera. The epithelial line was separated from the derma by dispase and MMP-9 expression was investigated by western blotting. Band (MW 92 kDa) corresponding to MMP-9 (d) appeared more intense in cell lysates from epidermis exposed to PV serum (lane 3), in comparison with those exposed to normal serum (*lane 2*) or control epidermis (*lane 1*). Figure was representative of three independent experiments.

We determined optimal conditions in pilot assays and than we carried out extensive experiments by incubating HaCaT cells with 3-fold concentrated 30% (v/v) PV and normal sera at selected time points. Western blot revealed that PV serum induced a sustained MMP-9 overexpression in keratinocytes if compared with control serum (Figure 1).

Up-regulation of the 92 kDa pro-MMP-9 became evident within 1h of incubation and reached the peak after 6h, keeping sustained expression after 12h as well. As expected, levels of the 82 kDa active MMP-9 were only slightly detectable, since MMP-9 is synthesized and secreted into its inactive form.

MMP-9 Overexpression in the Organ-Cuture Model of PV

Expression of MMP-9 was then investigated in epidermis from mouse organ cultures exposed to 3-fold concentrated 50% PV or normal serum. In our experimental conditions, PV serum was pathogenic as acantholysis occurs within 12 h (Figure 2. (a-c)). Thus, for the experiments, we incubated mouse organ cultures with sera for 12h.

After separation of the epithelial line from the underlying derma by dispase at 4°C, mouse epidermal keratinocyte cell lysates were probed for MMP-9 expression by western blotting. The intense up-regulation of keratinocyte MMP-9 was confirmed in the organ culture model of PV (Figure 2).

Taken together, results from *in vitro* studies on both keratinocyte monolayers and skin organ cultures revealed that MMP-9 is overexpressed is response to PV serum.

Secretion of MMP9 in Keratinocyte Intercellular Spaces Precedes Cell-Cell Detachment

MMP-9 expression on keratinocyte monolayers was then investigated by immunofluorescence microscopy. In normal conditions as well as in cells treated with normal serum, Texas red staining localized diffusely within the cells, and keratinocyte outlines were virtually indistinguishable by MMP-9 label (Figure 3). Conversely, MMP-9 staining appeared mainly localized on the surface of keratinocytes exposed to PV serum for 6h (Figure 4. (a)), compatible with its secretion within the intercellular spaces. Clearly, staining was not very intense, as the majority of extracellular MMP-9 was washed away during immunofluorescence procedures. The presumptive secretion of MMP-9 preceded the disruption of cell-cell contacts, occurring 24-48h after exposure to PV serum (not shown, see chapter 2). Indeed, by using PG to mark both cell periphery (linear staining) and intercellular adhesion areas (punctuate staining), keratinocytes showed no morphological changes and kept a punctuate membrane staining of FITC fluorescence (Figure 4. (b)), referred to as intact cell-cell adhesion structures. Overall, these data demonstrate that up-regulation MMP-9 represents an early event preceding acantholysis.

Secretion of MMP-9 in Culture Supernatants

To confirm that keratinocytes exposed to PV serum actually secrete MMP-9, we carried out a zymography assay on serum-free conditioned medium (SFCM). Cells were first incubated with 3-fold concentrated 30% PV or normal sera for 12h, then media were removed and replaced with fresh serum-free media. After 6h, the resulting SFCM were collected and zymography was assessed. Data showed a strong increase of gelatinolytic activity in SFCM from PV serum-treated cells, although the band corresponded to the 92 kDa pro-MMP-9, whereas the 82 kDa active MMP-9 appeared virtually undetectable in all samples (Figure 5).

These data confirmed that pro-MMP-9 is increasingly secreted by keratinocytes exposed to PV serum.

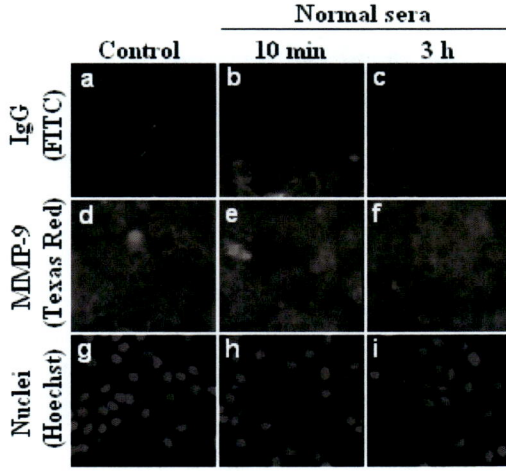

Figure 3. No staining of IgG was revealed on untreated or control sera-treated cells. MMP-9 localized diffusely within the cells.

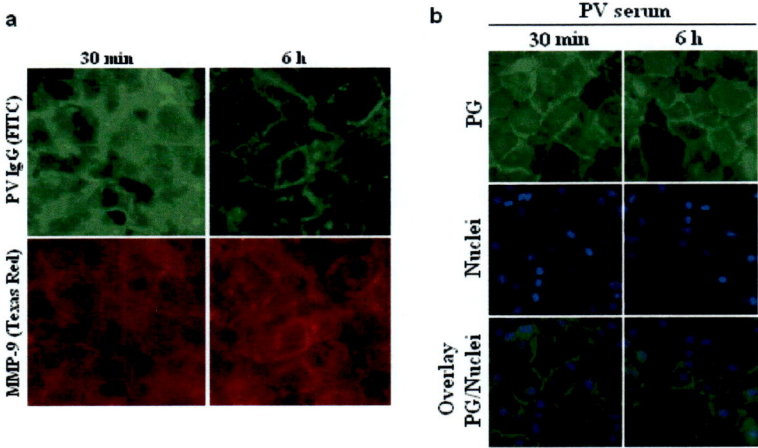

Figure 4. MMP-9 localizes within the inter-cellular spaces before disruption of cell-cell contacts. Immunofluorescence studies shows a diffuse Texas Red labelling 30 min after exposure to serum (a), corresponding to dramatic internalization of PV IgG (FITC staining). After 6 hours, Texas Red fluorescence, referred to as MMP-9, was mostly localized all around keratinocyte periphery. At point, however, sign of intercellular detachment were not recognized by neither PV IgG nor plakoglobin (PG) staining (b). Indeed, PG localized along cell membrane, suggesting that adhesion structures were yet integral. Figure was representative of at least two experiments conducted independently.

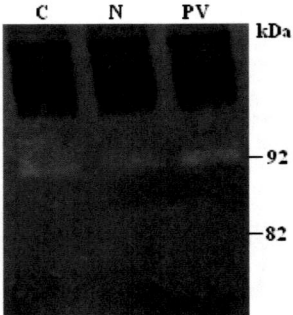

Figure 5. MMP-9 is secreted in culture supernatant of PV sera-treated cells. To assess whether MMP-9 overexpression is followed by its secretion within the extracellular compartment, 12 h SFCM of cultured keratinocytes previously treated with PV or normal sera, or untreated cells, were subjected to zymography. Gelatinolytic activity was detected in al samples, but SFCM from PV sera treated cells (PV, lane 3) showed an increase in the enzymatic activity compared with keratinocytes exposed to normal sera (N, lane 2) or untreated cells (C, lane 1). Triplicate experiments gave comparable results.

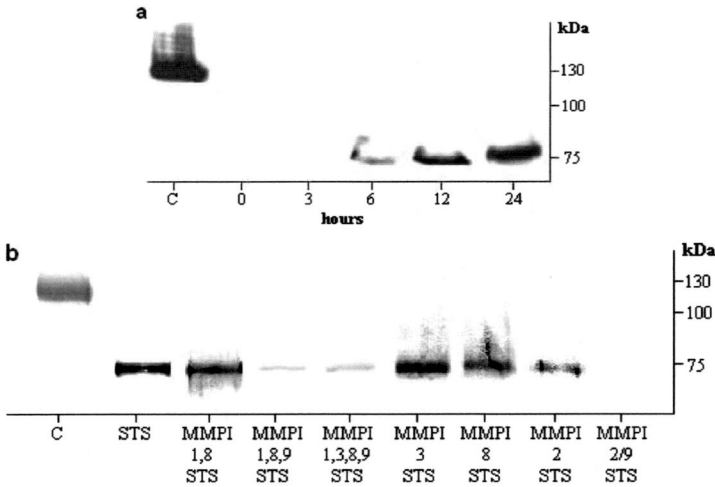

Figure 6. Extracellular cleavage of Dsg3 is blocked by MMP-9 inhibitors. Shedding of Dsg3 extracellular domain revealed by imunoblotting of the 100 fold-concentrated culture supernatant with the 5H10 antibody (a). Cells pretreated with MMPs inhibitors (b) at concentrations inhibiting MMP-9 showed a strong reduction of the 75 kDa extracellular domain of Dsg3 in culture supernatants (lane 4, 5 and 9). Cell culture supernatants were harvested 12 h after induction of apoptosis. Figures are representative of three independent.

Processing of Dsg3 by Gelatinases

One-day confluent cells were treated with 800nM STS. Changes in morphology, detachment from the substrate, DNA fragmentation and nuclear condensation demonstrated that HaCat cells responded to the apoptotic stimulus (not shown).

Appearance of fragmentation products concomitantly with decline of full-length Dsg3 from cell lysates is a well known evidence of proteolytic events against Dsg3 occurring during apoptosis [94]. Presence of a 75 kDa fragment of Dsg3 in culture supernatants (Figure 6. (a)) indicated that Dsg3 was proteolitically cleaved extracellularly during apoptotic pathways.

To investigate the role of specific MMPs involved in shedding Dsg3 from keratinocytes, we exposed cells to different concentrations of MMP inhibitors before the addition of staurosporine. MMPI-1 (80 and 200 µM) inhibited formation of the 75 kDa fragment of Dsg3, whereas MMPI-1 at lower concentrations or specific MMP3 and MMP8 inhibitors did not (Figure 6. (b, lanes 3-7)). These findings provide evidence that MMPI-1 reduces the cleavage of Dsg3 via inhibition of MMP-9. However, MMP-2 inhibition reduced the formation of the 75 kDa fragment (Figure 6. (b, lane 8)), suggesting a role for MMP-2 in the apoptotic cleavage of Dsg3. Consistently, inhibition of both MMP-2 and MMP-9 completely abolished the shedding of Dsg3 (Figure 6. (b, lane 9)). These data demonstrate that gelatinases activity is essential for the cleavage of Dsg3 in apoptotic keratinocytes.

Discussion

By means of Western blotting, zymography, and immunofluorescence analysis, in the present study we demonstrated for the first time that PV serum can induce sustained intracellular overexpression of proteinases such as MMP-9 followed by MMP-9 secretion. We have obtained evidence both *in vitro*, on keratinocyte monolayers and skin organ cultures, and *in vivo*, by establishing the neonatal mouse model of PV.

Despite morphological changes in keratinocytes became evident *in vitro* at least 24-48 after incubation with PV sera (our observations and those from refs 34 and 105), we found an increase in MMP-9 levels within 60-360 minutes, i.e. before cell-cell dyshesion were appreciated. Consistently, MMP-9 localization within intercellular spaces and its secretion in culture supernatant were demonstrated to occur before acantholysis took place, indicating that PV-induced changes in MMP-9 levels preceded the phenotypic manifestations of disease. Microarray analysis on the *in vivo* model of PV, which is reported in detail in chapter 8, showed significant transcriptional increase of a number of proteases, including MMPs which are known to digest E-cadherin and Dsg1 [143, 144]. Transcriptional up-regulation involved kallicrein as well. This finding is in keeping with previous studies which pointed out evidence of activation of the kinin system in plasma and blister content of patients with pemphigus. Also, kallikrein system is known to affect cytokeratin assembly and plasminogen activation, all potentially relevant events within the pathogenesis of PV acantholysis [145, 146]. For a long time, proteases such as plasmin have been considered as the actual effector of acantholysis in PV [147]. This hypothesis seemed setting when plasminogen knock-out mice were shown to develop blisters after injection with PV IgG [49]. However, the pathomechanisms occurring in PV patient's skin could be different from those triggered by highly concentrated PV IgG antibodies in the neonatal mouse model and, in any case, proteases other than plasmin could be involved in acantholysis. The ability of MMP-9 in cleaving Dsg3 during apoptosis [94] and its limited proteolytic spectrum in comparison to plasmin make MMP-9 the main candidate to investigate in the pathogenesis of PV acantholysis. Whether MMP-9 is proved being activated and cleaving Dsg3 in PV, then proteolytic theory and desmoglein compensation hypothesis should appear no more mutually exclusive (see below: *specific proteolysis hypothesis*). MMP-9 has been shown to play a crucial role in the pathogenesis of bullous pemphigoid, an autoimmune skin disease characterized by subepithelial blistering [148]. Indeed, MMP-9 knockout mice were resistant to experimental bullous pemphigoid and plasmin seemed to mediate the activation of MMP-9 in the early stages of disease. However, data reported by Liu et al. [148] also suggested that a plasmin-independent pathway was able to produce the activation of MMP-9 in later stages (24h-72h after mice injection), leading to lesion formation as well. Since plasminogen knockout mice develop blisters in the neonatal mouse model of PV, thus suggesting that plasmin is not directly involved in acantholysis, the alternative pathway leading to MMP-9 activation could play a major role in experimental PV.

The Specific Proteolysis Hypothesis

In light of our findings, we have proposed a novel explanation for PV pathogenesis [149]. Our hypothesis is based on the well-established different proteolytic spectrum of a series of metalloproteinases (MMP) shown to be involved in the disruption of keratinocyte adhesion structures. For example, members of the ADAM (a disintegrin and metallopeptidase) family of MMP have been shown to mediate the proteolysis of cell adhesion molecules such as E-cadherin and Dsg1 [143, 144], whereas Dsg3 is digested by enzymes belonging to the typical MMP family during apoptosis [141]. These findings are of great interest, given the well known ability of PV serum to induce apoptosis in keratinocytes both *in vitro* and *in vivo* [35, 111]. In particular, MMP-9 resulted the main executioner of Dsg3 in apoptotic keratinocytes [94]. Consistently, we have shown that MMP-9 is upregulated in response to PV serum (Figure 1). Furthermore, studies reported in chapter 4 demonstrate that Dsg3 undergoes proteolytic processing after exposure of keratinocytes to PV serum. Indeed, reduction of full-length Dsg3 paralleled with appearance of a proteolytic fragment encompassing the extracellular domain of Dsg3 (chapter 4, Figure 7). Overall, these findings strongly suggest that Dsg3 is targeted by proteases in response to PV serum, although the precise nature of this cleavage need to be further investigated. Hence, we propose that PV serum could induce secretion of MMP having differential specificity against cell adhesion molecules. In particular, Dsg1 and Dsg3 could be cleaved by either ADAM or typical MMP, respectively. Whether our hypothesis were demonstrated to be well-grounded, one can speculate that a subset of PV patients develop prevalently mucosal lesions because a specific spectrum of cell adhesion proteins becomes digested by a given protease, while cutaneous involvement takes place when the "compensating" action of yet unaffected adhesion molecules is targeted by other specific proteolytic enzymes. This should bring together both the proteolytic and desmoglein compensation theories.

Beyond Anti-Desmoglein Autoimmunity

Another intriguing conceptual implication is that the activation of specific MMP pathways is not necessarily related to the anti-desmoglein autoimmunity. On the contrary, we hypothesize that desmoglein-targeting antibodies could arise as a result of the proteolysis of cell-surface desmogleins by MMPs with subsequent release of their fragments within the intercellular spaces or diffusion outside the epithelium. With regard to this, it is worth of note that a rapid change in the strength of an antigenic stimulus is able to initiate a response in T cells [150]. Consistently, we have recently found the systemic 30-kDa fragment of Dsg3 (sDsg3) to physiologically occur in normal human serum, suggesting that peptide diffusion from the epidermis to the blood is not infrequent [114]. More interestingly, our recent discoveries demonstrate that pemphigus autoimmunity is just not restricted to keratinocytes, as PV IgG can target peripheral blood mononuclear cell antigen(s) [9]. Our provocative claims stem from the biologically well-grounded doubt that the deficit of Dsg3 alone cannot account for the disruption of epithelial integrity and blister formation. May so many proteins with adhesion function, such as Dsg1, Dsg2, Dsg4, desmocollins (Dsc1-3), and classical cadherins, altogether be unable to maintain cell-cell adhesion and compensate for the loss of Dsg3? This presumptive indispensability of Dsg3 is paradoxical, as most authors were not able to convincingly demonstrate the adhesive capacity of the Dsg3 *in vitro* (39-41). Moreover, inactivation of the Dsg3 gene or depletion of Dsg3 from keratinocytes within mouse epidermis or in cultured monolayers failed to induce gross skin blistering or disrupt desmosomes, respectively [42, 73, 151].

In summary, we have reported that PV serum induces MMP-9 overexpression both in keratinocyte monolayers and skin organ culture, followed by its secretion in the culture medium. Evidence of proteinase upregulation was also observed in the neonatal mouse model of PV. Further studies will address whether MMP-9 plays a pathogenic role in the induction of acantholysis. The specific proteolysis theory proposed by us is not just a return to the past. It suggests that proteases such as MMPs may specifically cleave well defined clusters of cell-adhesion proteins, including desmogleins. On the basis of the current knowledge on MMP substrate specificity, we propose that Dsg1 and Dsg3, together with other important cadherins, could be cleaved by either ADAM or typical MMPs, respectively. This should be compatible with the compensation theory viewed as a more extended concept, although we cannot exclude that anti-desmoglein autoimmunity arises just after PV lesions have developed. Our research group is intensely working on these ideas to investigate the putative involvement of MMPs in pemphigus. Whether the causal role of MMPs will be substantiated by consistent findings, then new non-steroideal therapeutic strategies could be available to treat this serious disease.

Chapter 8

Microarray Analysis of Diseased Tissues: Cell Adhesion Is Down-Regulated on the Gene Level in Pemphigus

Since complex alterations are induced in keratinocytes by PV serum, screening of transcriptional changes could be an interesting approach to understand PV pathophysiology.

Here we have shown by microarray analysis that PV sera induced multiple changes in gene expression and regulatory events involve both kinases and several adhesion molecules. We have obtained evidence both *in vitro*, on keratinocyte monolayers and skin organ cultures, and *in vivo*, by establishing the neonatal mouse model of PV.

Microarray analysis on keratinocytes detected that PV serum induced important changes in genes coding for one and the same proteins with known biological functions involved in PV disease (560 differentially expressed genes were identified).

In vivo PV serum was found to alter multiple different pathways by microarray analysis (1463 differentially expressed genes were identified). The most significantly enriched pathways were cell communication, gap junction, focal adhesion, adherens junction, and tight junction. This alteration may influence the evolution of PV and its therapy.

Introduction

Although it has become clear that acantholysis is not just the result of a direct steric hindrance between IgG and Dsg3, it is not yet clear how does PV serum affect the regulation of cell adhesion strength in keratinocytes. Indeed, while phosphorylation events occur to rapidly regulate protein activity, changes in gene expression take place slower but they are expression of a stable response of the cell to the external clues. Here, in order to define disease mechanisms, we took an empirical unbiased approach analyzing keratinocytes and mice skin treated with PV by large genome microarray technologies. Our data indicate a deregulation of transcripts primarily involved in cell organization and structure of epithelial tissue and keratins.

The development of several gene expression profiling methods, such as comparative genomic hybridization (CGH), differential display, serial analysis of gene expression (SAGE), and gene microarray, together with the sequencing of the human genome, has provided an opportunity to monitor and investigate the complex cascade of molecular events. The availability of such large amounts of information has shifted the attention of scientists towards a nonreductionist approach to biological phenomena. High throughput technologies can be used to follow changing patterns of gene expression over time. Among them, gene microarray has become prominent because it is easier to use, does not require large-scale DNA sequencing, and allows for the parallel quantification of thousands of genes from multiple samples. Gene microarray technology is rapidly spreading worldwide and has the potential to drastically change the therapeutic approach to patients

Microarray analysis results in the gathering of massive amounts of information concerning gene expression profiles of different cells and experimental conditions. Here, we used this novel technology to screen gene expression changes both in *in vitro* and *in vivo* models of PV.

Materials and Methods

Passive Transfer of Sera in Neonatal Mice

This study was conducted according to the Guidelines for Animal Experiments of the American Heart Association and rules of the National Institutes of Health (NIH publication No. 85-23, revised 1985). Eight to twelve-hour-old neonatal balb/c mice were injected intraperitoneally through a 30-gauge needle with 150μl 10-fold concentrated sera. Some pups were pretreated with 100μg/g roscovitine in 20μl PBS (n=6) or 20μl PBS as a control (n=6). After 12 hours, the animals were subjected to gentle scraping of the lumbar skin to induce eventually the Nikolskiy phenomenon, then, 24 hours after injection, mice were evaluated for macroscopic blistering. Biopsies were taken by perilesional areas, if any, by using a standard 5 mm skin biopsy punch. After rinsing in PBS, these skin samples were either stored at -80°C and subsequently subjected to RNA extraction or immediately fixed in 10% formalin for regular histological analysis.

Cell Cultures and Treatments

We have exposed cultured cells to PV patient sera as proposed in chapter 2. Primary human keratinocytes were isolated from tongue specimens of patients undergoing glossoplasty as detailed. HaCaT cells were maintained in DMEM enriched with 10% FBS and 1% antibiotics/antimycotic, as described (chapter 2). Primary keratinocytes and HaCaT were growth at 37°C in an atmosphere humidified with 5% CO_2. At the time of the experiment, cells were seeded on 35mm Petri plastic dishes and growth to confluence. Keratinocytes were treated as specified in the Results section.

RNA Extraction, Microarrays Analysis, and RT-PCR

Tissues were snap-frozen in liquid nitrogen and stored at −80°C until use. Total RNAs were extracted from mouse tissues and cultured cells using Trizol^{TM} solution (Invitrogen), according to the manufacturer's instructions. The integrity of the RNA was assessed by denaturing agarose gel electrophoresis (virtual presence of sharp 28S and 18S bands) and spectrophotometry. 5μg total RNA was used as starting material for the cDNA preparation. The first and second strand cDNA synthesis was performed using the GeneChip One-Cycle cDNA Synthesis Kit (Affymetrix) according to the manufacturers instructions. Labeled cRNA was prepared using the GeneChip IVT Labeling Kit (Affymetrix) according to the manufacturers instructions. Following the IVT reaction, the unincorporated nucleotides were removed using RNeasy columns (Qiagen). 15 μg of cRNA was for hybridization onto the Affymetrix Mouse Genome 430A 2.0 and Affymetrix Human Genome

U133 2.0 probe array cartridge. The washing and staining procedure was performed in the Affymetrix Fluidics Station 450. The probe arrays were scanned at 560 nm using a confocal laser-scanning microscope (GeneChip® Scanner 3000). The readings from the quantitative scanning were analyzed by the Affymetrix Gene Expression Analysis Software. RNA was reverse transcribed with Superscript III (Invitrogen) using 1µg total RNA and 100 ng random primers. Primer sequences and corresponding PCR conditions are found in the literature. Results were normalized to GAPDH, used as a housekeeping gene. We used a glyceraldehydes-3-phophate deydrogenase (gapdh)-specific fragment to verify the integrity of the RNA preparation. The intensity of the amplified bands was quantified by densitometry and referred to that obtained with gapdh (Quantity One, Bio-Rad).

Ontology Assessment

We subjected the list of differentially expressed transcripts to gene ontology using DAVID (Database for Annotation, Visualization and Integrated Discovery), Web-based applications (http://david.abcc.ncifcrf.gov) that allow access to a relational database of functional annotation [152].

Results

Modulation of Gene Expression by PV Sera in Keratinocytes Detected by DNA Microarray

The cRNA generated from a pool of 3 different mRNA estraction (a mean of 2 different experiments, each in duplicate) for each condition (keratinocytes with normal serum, keratinocytes with PV serum) and arrays contained 14,500 well-characterized human genes (22,215 total genes comprehensive of EST sequences) were used to measure effects of treatments of keratinocytes with PV serum *versus* normal serum. Only genes that have the threshold of 50 arbitrary detection unit and absolute fold change (FC) value greater than 1 have been included in the complete lists of genes. The FC value in a gene expression can be calculated as $FC = 2^{[Signal\ Log\ Ratio\ (SLR)]}$. The SLR algorithm measures the magnitude and direction of change between transcript levels of the experimental and baseline chips. The use of logs in the analysis between the probe sets eliminates difficulties caused by one very high data point in the set masking information from lower valued data points. Base 2 is used as the log scale, therefore a SLR of 1 represents a two-fold increase in abundance of an mRNA and a value of –1 represents a two-fold reduction in transcript expression. Of course, we did not considered in those lists genes corresponding to control probes. Overall, PV serum decreased transcription of *231* genes and increased transcription of *329* genes. Important changes were observed in transcription of the genes coding for different proteins with known biological functions as follws: 1) components of cell organization and structure (trasgelin, keratin 13, keratin 6A); 2) cells adhesion molecules (laminin gamma 2, Rho family GTPase 3, cadherin 4, claudin 7, epithelial V-like antigen 1, protocadherin gamma subfamily C 3); 3) regulators of progression through cell cycle and apoptosis (CDC-like kinase 1, fibroblast growth factor 2, interleukin 1 beta, vascular endothelial growth factor B, CD70 molecule); 4) cell signaling proteins (follistain, Rho-guanine nucleotide exchange factor, stanniocalcin 2); 5) enzymes involved in general cellular metabolism (uridine phosphorylase 1, matrix metallopeptidase 14, prostaglandin E). These and other genes are listed in Table III. To validate data obtained by microarray analysis, we performed PCR on differentially expressed genes. The levels of induction detected by RT-PCR were similar to those observed on the microarrays (data not show).

These screening experiments confirmed a previous study [135] where IgG isolated from PV patients were used, although the use of PV serum showed a larger number of up-regulated genes.

Evidence that cdk2 Inhibition through Roscovitine Prevents Acantholysis in the Neonatal Mouse Model of PV

Since cdk2 overxpression was the most remarkable phenomenon seen in the present study, 8-12-hour-old neonatal balb/c mice were injected intraperitoneally through a 30-gauge needle with 150 l 10-fold concentrated PV (n=4) or control sera (n=2). All mice receiving PV serum, but not control serum, developed skin blisters approximately 24 hours after a single injection. The blisters resulted from suprabasilar acantholysis, as revealed by histological examination (Figure 2. (e), *normal serum and PV serum*). The passive transfer study was carried out in the presence of roscovitine, a well known inhibitor of cdk2 activity (33). 100 μg roscovitine per g of body weight dissolved in 20 μl PBS (n=6) or 20μl PBS as a control (n=6, not shown) were administered intraperitoneally 2 h before the i.p. injection of different PV sera.

Remarkably, under our experimental conditions, none of mice (n=6) pretreated with roscovitine developed any skin lesion, both clinically and histologically (Figure 2(e), *roscovitine pre-treatment followed by PV serum*) within 24 h after i.p. injection with PV sera (n=4).

Modulation of Gene Expression by PV Sera in Mouse Skin Lesions Detected by DNA Microarray

To elucidate the molecular mechanism of roscovitine action on mice treated with PV serum, cRNA was generated from a pool of different mRNA isolated from skin samples of mice (n=6). In this experiment we have decided to use PV serum. In pilot array study on keratinocytes, we determined that PV serum induced important changes in transcription of the genes coding for one and the same proteins with known biological functions involved in PV disease. Arrays contained 14,000 well-characterized mouse genes (22,000 total genes comprehensive of EST sequences) were used to measure effects of treatments of mice with PV serum *versus* normal serum, PV serum in presence of roscovitine *versus* PV serum and PV serum in presence of roscovitine *versus* normal serum. In this case we have considered only genes that have the threshold of 50 arbitrary detection unit and absolute fold change value greater or equal than 2 have been included in the complete lists of genes. Overall, PV serum decreased transcription of *1114* genes and increased transcription of *349* genes. Roscovitine modified the gene expression profile in the presence of PV serum. Compared with the effect of PV serum alone, exposure to PV serum in presence of roscovitine showed up-regulation of *117* genes and down-regulation of *153* genes, using the same filter criteria adopted for the comparison of PV serum versus normal serum. Additionally, some genes down-regulated or up-regulated in the presence of PV serum alone were up-regulated or down-regulated respectively when treated with roscovitine (ie, plakophilin 3, jagged 2, and calpain 6) (Table 2).

The biological process ontology and KEGG pathway terms associated with the differentially expressed genes were examined using the online available DAVID bioinformatics database. The reciprocal changes were observed in transcription of the genes coding for proteins with known biological functions as follows: 1) components of cell organization and structure (keratins, transglutaminase, and involucrin); 2) cells adhesion molecules (jagged 2, desmoplakin, bystin-like, reelin, and calpain 6); 3) regulators of cell cycle progression (cyclin-dependent kinase 8, cyclin D1, cyclin D2, and cyclin G associated kinase; 5) cell death (cyclin-dependent kinase inhibitor 1A (P21), Fas death domain-associated protein, and growth arrest specific 1); 6) defense response (CD93 antigen, and histocompatibility 2, D region); 7) immuno response (histocompatibility 2, D region locus 1, and Interferon activated gene 203). As usual, to validate data obtained by microarray analysis, we performed PCR on several differentially expressed genes involved in cell communication pathways. The levels of induction detected by RT-PCR were similar to those observed on the microarrays.

Shared Microarray Results

Comparing results from both human and mice microarrays, different genes were down-regulated and up-regulated. The changes were observed in transcription of the genes coding for proteins involved in the same biological functions, such as cell adhesion, cytoskeleton organization and biogenesis, regulation of progression through cell cycle.

Table 1. Gene expression of keratinocytes treated with pemphigus vulgaris serum *versus* normal serum (PVS *vs* NS). The results are expressed as both the signal log ratio (SLR) and the direction of the change, i.e. an increase (I), a decrease (D)

Representative Public ID	Gene title	Gene Ontology (Biological Process)	PVS *vs* NS (SLR)	Chromosomal Location
NM_006350	follistatin	cell regulation and signaling	1.42 D	chr5
NM_002421	Matrix metallopeptidase 1 (interstitial collagenase)	Peptidoglycan metabolism	1.06 D	chr11
NM_003186	transgelin	Cytoskeleton organization and biogenesis	0.98 D	chr11
NM_002658	Plasminogen activator, urokinase	proteolysis	0.88 D	chr10
AI251890	CDC-like kinase 1	regulation of progression through cell cycle	0.87 D	chr2

Table 1. (Continued)

Representative Public ID	Gene title	Gene Ontology (Biological Process)	PVS vs NS (SLR)	Chromosomal Location
NM_022448	Rho-guanine Nucleotide exchange factor	Intracellular signaling cascade	0.86 D	chr5
AF116771	tumor protein p73-like	Skeletal development	0.81 D	chr3
NM_001924	growth arrest and DNA-damage inducible, alpha	regulation of cyclin dependent protein kinase activity	0.76 D	chr1
NM_018891	laminin, gamma2	cell adhesion	0.73 D	chr1
NM_003364	Uridine Phosphorylase 1	Nucleoside metabolism	0.73 D	chr7
NM_003856	interleukin 1 receptor like 1	DNA methylation	0.73 D	chr2
AV700298	CD44 molecule (Indian blood group)	ureteric bud branching	0.70 D	chr11
NM_006290	tumor necrosis factor, alpha-induced protein3	ubiquitin cycle	0.69 D	chr6
NM_019885	Cytochrome P450, family 26, subfamily B, polypeptide 1	electron transport	0.69 D	chr2
AI738896	tumor necrosis factor, alpha-induced protein3	ubiquitin cycle	0.65 D	chr6
BG054844	Rho family GTPase 3	cell adhesion	0.63 D	chr2
M27968	Fibroblast growth factor 2 (basic)	regulation of progression through cell cycle	0.62 D	chr4

Representative Public ID	Gene title	Gene Ontology (Biological Process)	PVS vs NS (SLR)	Chromosomal Location
U82828	Ataxia telangiectasia mutated (includes complementatin groups A, C and D)	DNA repair	0.62 D	chr11
AL096842	Mitochondrial Tumor suppressor 1	Unknown	0.59 D	chr8
NM_014709	Ubiquitin specific peptidase 34	Ubiquitin Dependent Protein catabolism	0.57 D	chr2
AI435828	stanniocalcin 2	cell surface receptor linked signal transduction	0.56 D	chr5
AL110158	Calmodulin regulated spectrin associated protein 1-like 1	Unknown	0.56 D	chr1
BE786164	Activating transcription factor 2	transcription	0.54 D	chr2
NM_024883	cadherin 4, type 1, R cadherin (retinal)	cell adhesion	0.52 D	chr20
NM_001307	claudin 7	Calcium independent cell cell adhesion	0.52 D	chr17
U77914	jagged 1 (Alagille syndrome)	angiogenesis	0.51 D	chr20
M15330	interleukin 1, beta	regulation of progression through cell cycle	0.50 D	chr2
NM_022969	Fibroblast growth factor receptor 2 (keratinocyte growth factor receptor)	protein amino acid phosphorylation	0.50	chr10

Table 1. (Continued)

Representative Public ID	Gene title	Gene Ontology (Biological Process)	PVS vs NS (SLR)	Chromosomal Location
BC000305	caspase 6, apoptosis-related cysteine peptidase	proteolysis	0.50 I	chr4
D50683	Transforming growth factor, beta receptor II (70/80kDa)	protein amino acid phosphorylation	0.50 I	chr3
NM_002730	protein kinase, cAMP dependent, catalytic, alpha	Mesoderm formation	0.52 I	chr19
NM_005797	epithelial V-like antigen 1	cell adhesion	0.54 I	chr11
AF031469	Major Histocompatibilty complex, class I related	Antigen processing and presentation of peptide antigen via MHC class I	0.55 I	chr1q
NM_004292	Ras and Rab Interactor 1	endocytosis	0.56 I	chr11
AI762811	mitogen-activated protein kinase kinase 2	protein amino acid phosphorylation	0.58 I	chr19
W47179	cathepsin B	Proteolysis	0.59 I	chr8
AI359368	Leucine zipper EF hand containing transmembrane protein 1	Signal transduction	0.64 I	chr4
NM_001252	CD70 molecule	apoptosis	0.66 I	chr19
NM_014624	S100 calcium binding protein A6	regulation of progression through cell cycle	0.66 I	chr1
NM_001191	BCL2-like 1	anti-apoptosis	0.67 I	chr20

Representative Public ID	Gene title	Gene Ontology (Biological Process)	PVS vs NS (SLR)	Chromosomal Location
U13698	caspase 1, apoptosis related cysteine peptidase (interleukin 1, beta, convertase)	proteolysis	0.68 I	chr11
NM_003730	ribonuclease T2	RNA catabolism	0.69 I	chr6
BC006439	Protocadherin gamma subfamily C, 3	cell adhesion	0.72 I	chr5
NM_000043	Fas (TNF receptor superfamily, member 6)	protein complex assembly	0.74 I	chr10
NM_005345	heat shock 70kDa protein 1A	protein folding	0.85 I	chr6
NM_004995	Matrix Metallopeptidase 14 (membrane inserted)	Peptidoglycan metabolism	0.86 I	chr14q
NM_014316	calcium regulated heat stable protein 1,24kDa	regulation of transcription, DNA-dependent	0.86 I	chr16
NM_005951	Metallothionein 1H	UNKNOW	0.87 I	chr16
NM_003377	Vascular endothelial growth factor B	regulation of progression through cell cycle	0.89 I	chr11
NM_005983	S-phase kinase associated protein 2 (p45)	regulation of progression through cell cycle	0.89 I	chr5
NM_002274	keratin 13	Epidermis development	0.98 I	chr17
AI675178	calcium channel, voltage dependent, gamma subunit 4	ion transport	1.2 I	chr17
NM_004878	prostaglandin E synthase	Prostaglandin metabolism	1.4 I	chr9
AL569511	keratin 6A	Ectoderm development	1.46 I	chr12

Table 2. Gene expression of samples treated with pemphigus vulgaris serum *versus* normal serum (PVS *vs* NS), The results are expressed as both the signal log ratio (SRL) and the direction of the change, i.e. an increase (I), a decrease (D). or no differential expression (NDE)

Representative Public ID	Gene title	Gene Ontology (Biological Process)	PVS *vs* NS (SLR)	Chromos Location
D89901	keratin associated protein 6-3	Unknown	4.3D	chr16
NM_054097	Phosphatidylinositol 4-phosphate 5-kinase, type II, gamma	Unknown	4.3D	chr10
NM_016879	keratin complex 2, basic, gene 18	Unknown	7.0D	chr15
NM_009387	thymidine kinase 1	DNA replication	5.0D	chr11
NM_010666	keratin complex-1, acidic, gene C29	Cytoskeleton organization and biogenesis	7.5D	chr1
NM_025276	envoplakin	keratinization	4.7D	chr11
BB283187	carnitine O octanoyltransferase	Lipid metabolism	5.5D	chr5
NM_016705	kinesin family member 21A	Microtubule based process	3.5D	chr15
BC019374	glutamate-cysteine ligase, catalytic subunit	Glutathione biosynthesis	5.1D	chr9
BC027245	gamma-aminobutyric acid (GABA-A) receptor, pi	transport	4.0D	chr11
NM_010659	keratin complex 1, acidic, gene 1	Cytoskeleton Organization and biogenesis	8.5D	chr1
NM_010864	myosin Va	Cytoskeleton Organization and biogenesis	4.2D	chr9
AK005226	calcium binding protein 39	Unknown	3.4D	chr1
BC025618	ATPase, Na+/K+ transporting, alpha 1 polypeptide	Transport	2.0D	chr3
NM_134131	tumor necrosis factor, alpha-induced rotein8	Unknown	3.3D	chr18
BC024835	structure specific recognition protein 1	regulation of transcription, DNA dependent	3.2D	chr2

Representative Public ID	Gene title	Gene Ontology (Biological Process)	PVS vs NS (SLR)	Chromos Location
BM208103	Cytoskeleton associated protein 2	Unknown	3.2D	chr8
NM_022886	sciellin	Epidermis development	2.6D	chr14
NM_008631	metallothionein 4	Electron transport	5.8D	chr8
AF083876	epithelial membrane protein 2	Unknown	3.7D	chr16
BG079188	bystin-like	cell adhesion	2.7D	chr1
NM_012006	acyl-CoA thioesterase 1	long-chain fatty acid metabolism	2.6D	chr12
AF296657	ubiquitin-conjugating enzyme E2G 2	Protein modification	2.3D	chr10
BM119387	villin 2	regulation of cell shape	3.3D	chr17
NM_007991	fibrillarin	rRNA processing	1.8D	chr7
NM_009983	cathepsin D	proteolysis	2.2D	chr7
AK020708	glycoprotein, synaptic 21	Unknown	3.3D	chr8
X75650	keratin complex 1, acidic, gene 3	Cytoskeleton Organization and biogenesis	7.4D	chr11
AA727386	keratin associated protein 8-1	Unknown	6.8D	chr16
NM_009257	serine (or cysteine) peptidase inhibitor, clade B, member 5	Unknown	6.4D	chr1
NM_011060	peptidyl arginine deiminase, type III	Protein modification	6.0D	chr4
AF087470	S100 calcium binding protein A3	Electron transport	4.9D	chr3
X00246	histocompatibility 2, D region locus 1	Immune response	4.4D	chr17
BC004663	Desmocollin 2	cell adhesion	4.5D	chr18
AI506986	gasdermin 1	Unknown	4.6D	chr11
BC026422	transglutaminase 1, K polypeptide	Protein modification	4.1D	chr14
BC026051	laminin, beta 2	Electron transport	3.8D	chr9
BB006219	tyrosinase-related protein 1	Melanin Biosynthesis from tyrosine	3.4D	chr4

Table 2. (Continued)

Representative Public ID	Gene title	Gene Ontology (Biological Process)	PVS vs NS (SLR)	Chromos Location
M98547	receptor-like tyrosine kinase	protein amino acid phosphorylation	3.2D	chr9
BI410170	ribonuclease T2	Unknown	3.0D	chr17
AA798563	keratin complex 1, acidic, gene 17	Cellular morphogenesis	2.5D	chr11
AW475993	plakophilin 3	cell adhesion	2.0D	chr7
AV241768	tumor-associated calcium signal transducer 2	Defense response	2.0D	chr6
BC014783	Proteasome (prosome, macropain) subunit, beta type 3	Ubiquitin Dependent Protein catabolism	1.5D	chr11
NM_009140	chemokine (C-X-C motif) ligand 2	chemotaxis	4.4I	chr5
NM_010516	cysteine rich protein 61	regulation of cell growth	3.2I	chr53
NM_007429	angiotensin II receptor, type 2	Angiotensin Mediated Vasodilation During regulation of blood pressure	3.2I	chrX
BB241535	suppressor of cytokine signaling 3	regulation of cell growth	2.7I	chr11
AV026617	FBJ osteosarcoma oncogene	regulation of progression through cell cycle	3.9I	chr12
BB238025	ZXD family zinc finger C	Unknow	5.2I	chr6
NM_009398	tumor necrosis factor alpha induced protein 6	cell adhesion	6.8I	chr2
NM_011993	Dihydropyrimidinase like 4	Unknow	6.5I	chr7
AY027660	hornerin	development	6.1I	chr3
BB225239	Interleukin 10 receptor, alpha	cell surface receptor linked signal transduction	6.0	chr9
BC026555	kallikrein B, plasma 1	proteolysis	3.8I	chr8

Representative Public ID	Gene title	Gene Ontology (Biological Process)	PVS vs NS (SLR)	Chromos Location
NM_011261	reelin	Cellular Morphogenesis During differentiation	3.0I	chr5
AI747133	calpain 6	Cellular Morphogenesis During differentiation	2.4I	chrX
BI794771	procollagen, type I, alpha 1	Phosphate transport	2.0I	chr11

Discussion

Here we have shown by microarray analysis that PV sera induced multiple changes in gene expression and regulatory events involve both kinases and several adhesion molecules. We have obtained evidence both *in vitro*, on keratinocyte monolayers and skin organ cultures, and *in vivo*, by establishing the neonatal mouse model of PV.

Different genes downregulated in keratinocites PV serum-treated were also downregulated in another study wherein isolated IgG from PV patients were used [135]. Noteworthy, the use of PV serum showed a larger number of up-regulated genes. The microarray that we designed on mice skin treated with PV serum was intended to evaluate the expression of know and unknown genes by comparing the gene expression with the response to PV serum.

Keratins are major structural proteins in epithelial cells. They make up the largest subgroup of intermediate filament proteins and form a dynamic network of 10-12 nm filaments, built type I/type II heterodimers, in the cytoplasm of epithelial cells [153]. A major function of keratin is to protect epithelial cells from mechanical and non-mechanical stresses that cause cell rupture and death [154, 155]. We have found several genes encoding components of intracellular desmosome junction. Desmosomes together with adherens junction represent the major adherens cell-cell junctions of epithelial cells. Both types of junctions are connected with the cytoskeleton and represent sites of mechanical coupling between cells. In contrast to adherens junctions, which are linked to actin micro filament system, desmosome are associated with intermediate filaments. Moreover, we have found PV serum induced down-regulation of different desmosomal cadherins such as desmocollin 2, desmoglein 2.

Keratinocytes grown in low Ca^{2+} medium proliferate but do not form cell-cell contacts. A rise in Ca^{2+} concentration induces rapid assembly of adherens junctions and desmosomes. Variations in Ca^{2+} concentration seem to interfere with normal desmosome assembly. Therefore, changes in intracellular Ca^{2+} concentration may induce regulatory signal [156]. This putative role of Ca^{2+} in keratinocyte signaling leading to acantholysis is consistent with the finding that PV autoimmunity targets acetycholine receptors (AChR) [81]. In fact, PV patients develop autoantibodies against the α9 AChR Ca^{2+} channel with dual, muscarinic and nicitic activity which regulates epidermal adhesion [25]. Interestingly, we found in the present study an up-regulation (calcium channel, voltage-dependent, L type, alpha 1D subunit) and down-regulation (gap junction membrane channel protein alpha 1) of genes involved in calcium transport. In addition, cell signaling induced by the non-desmoglein autoantibodies produced by PV patients that may target keratinocyte AChR modulates Src and EGF receptor kinase, which have been shown to play an important role in regulation of intracellular adhesion [157]. Moreover, we have found (see chapter 5) that PV IgG can recognize an antigen other than desmoglein 3 on peripheral blood mononuclear cell surface [9]. Interestingly, we found an up-regulation of inflammatory cytokines previously reported to be involved in PV acantholysis, such as TNF and IL-10 30, 31].

Another intriguing finding of our study is given by the changes of gene expression by microarray analysis on the *in vivo* model of PV showed a significant transcriptional increase of a number of proteases in addition to a marked reduction of several components of the keratinocyte adhesion structures. Among others, it should be noted that a member of the ADAM (a disintegrin and metallopeptidase) family of MMP displayed a 4-fold increase (table 2). This is of particular interest because ADAM proteases have been shown to mediate the proteolysis of cell adhesion molecules such as E-cadherin and Dsg1 [143, 144]. Microarray data also showed kallikrein, a serum proteinases synthesized to a major extent by the liver as an inactive enzyme, to be almost 5-fold upregulated in epidermis of PV sera-injected mice (table 2). This finding is relevant to our model of acantholysis, as kallikrein system is known to affect cytokeratin assembly and plasminogen activation [145, 146].

In conclusion, microarray analysis of diseased tissues in experimental models of PV shed light on the molecular pathways involved in acantholysis.

Chapter 9

Pharmacological Block of Acantholysis: Towards Novel Therapies for the Treatment of Pemphigus

Autoantibodies present in PV patients can promote detrimental effects by triggering altered transduction of signals which results in a final acantholysis. We have previously shown (chapter 6) that phopsphorylation events are impaired in PV and PV sera are able to promote cell cycle progression by inducing the accumulation of cyclin-dependent kinase 2 (cdk2). Here, we finally sought to assess the pathogenic role of cdk2 in acantholysis. We used further different approaches to investigate the actual role of cdk2. Pharmacological inhibition of cdk2 activity through roscovitine prevented blister formation and acantholysis in the mouse model of the disease. Major changes in gene expression induced by roscovitine were then studied through comparison effects of PV serum alone and in association with roscovitine. Interestingly, PV-dependent changes in gene regulation were abrogated by roscovitine, thus showing that cdk2 is crucial in orchestrating intracellular signalling which impair desmosome adhesion strength in pemphigus. Our data indicate that major cdk2-dependent multiple gene regulatory events are present in PV. This alteration may influence the evolution of PV and its therapy.

Taken together, the results presented here open new avenues for a non-steroideal treatment of pemphigus. Indeed, the molecular effects of PV can be targeted by using selective cdk2 inhibitors.

Introduction

In the previous chapters, we have dissected the crucial pathways involved in acantholysis. Posphorylation events have been shown to be triggered by PV serum in keratinocytes both *in vitro* and *in vivo*. Among the array of kinases which orchestrate the acantholytic cascade, cdk2 has shown a pivotal role. This evidence was obtained both in cultured cells and *in vivo*, by using skin biopsies of PV patients. We observed also that PV serum increased the cell cycle progression. Second, we revealed that silencing of cdk2 was able to reduce disruption of cell-cell contacts in keratinocytes exposed to PV serum (see chapter 5). Hence, we assumed that cdk2 is essential for PV acantholysis *in vitro*. Interestingly, in addition to rapid alterations in protein phosphorylation state, microarray analysis has revealed that PV serum acts on the transcriptional level by down-regulating cell-adhesion molecules. This is perfectly consistent with the fact that pemphigus is just a disease of intercellular adhesion. Finally, here we sought to assess the pathogenic role of cdk2 in acantholysis.

Materials and Methods

Passive Transfer of Sera in Neonatal Mice

The *in vitro* model of PV was established as detailed in chapter 2. Mouse skin samples were either stored at -80°C and subsequently subjected to RNA extraction or immediately fixed in 10% formalin for regular histological analysis.

Cell Cultures and Treatments

We have exposed cultured cells to PV patient sera as proposed in chapter 2. HaCaT cells were growth at 37°C in an atmosphere humidified with 5% CO_2. At the time of the experiment, cells were seeded on 35mm Petri plastic dishes and growth to confluence. Keratinocytes were treated as specified in the Results section.

RNA Extraction, Microarrays Analysis, RT-PCR, and Ontology Assessment

Tissues were snap-frozen in liquid nitrogen and stored at −80°C until use. Total RNAs were extracted from mouse tissues and cultured cells as detailed in chapter 8. RT-PCR and microarray analysis were carried out according to the protocols described in chapter 8.

The list of differentially expressed transcripts were subjected to gene ontology using DAVID application (chapter 8)

Standard Immunofluorescence Microscopy and Histology

Conventional immunofluorescence studies and histological analysis were carried out according to standard procedures (chapter 2).

Results

Inhibition of Phosphorylation Events Prevents Pemphigus Acantholysis

Since specific kinase activity was enhanced by serum of PV patients in keratinocytes, we blocked phosphorilation events with STS, a broad kinase inhibitor. Indeed, at the concentration used (100 nM), STS was able to decrease or abrogate the three PV-specific phosphorylation events whereas it does not induce apoptosis. When keratinocytes were incubated with STS along with 30% (v/v) PV serum for 48h, *in vitro* acantholysis was dramatically reduced, as shown by immunofluorescence images (Figure 1). Some cells affected by acantholytic dismorphisms were observed in the periphery of the colony (not shown).

No signs of nuclear condensation were observed (Figure 1. (g,h)), confirming that neither 30% PV serum alone nor in addition to low concentration (100 nM) STS do trigger nuclear condensation.

On the contrary, cycloheximide and momensin, which inhibit protein synthesis and lysosomal degradation, respectively, did not prevent acantholysis of cells exposed to PV serum (Figure 1. (d,e)). These results overall demonstrated that abrogation of PV-specific protein phosphorilation prevents cell-cell detachment and acantholysis.

Evidence that cdk2 Inhibition through Roscovitine Prevents Acantholysis in the Neonatal Mouse Model of PV

Since cdk2 overxpression was the most remarkable phenomenon seen in the present study, 8-12-hour-old neonatal balb/c mice were injected intraperitoneally through a 30-gauge needle with 150 l 10-fold concentrated PV (n=4) or control sera (n=2).

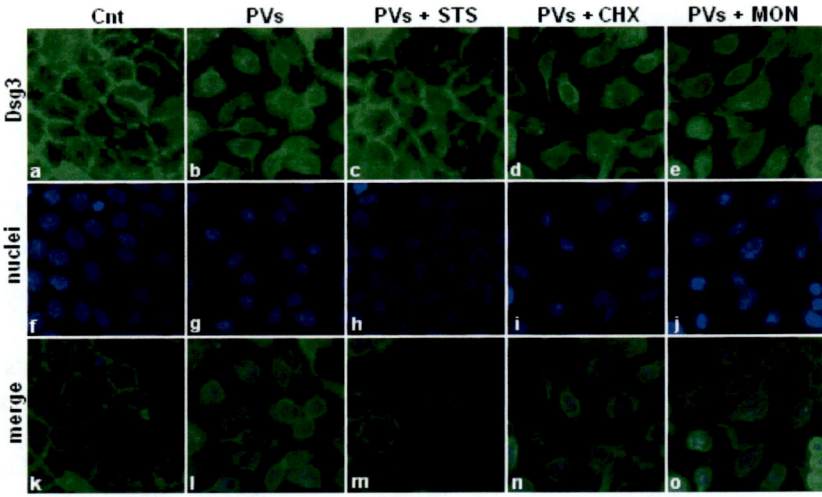

Figure 1. Central The cells were analyzed by indirect immunofluorescence double-staining with anti-desmoglein 3 (5H10) antibody (FITC-conjugated, green) and DAPI (blue). Individual color images were combined for visualization of an overlay image (merge). Cells preincubated with either cycloheximide (CHX) (d, i) or monensin (MON) (e, j) in addition to PV serum (48 hrs) exhibited features virtually undistinguishable from those seen in cells exposed solely to PV serum (b, g). Keratinocytes detached from one another, Dsg3 underwent dramatic redistribution. FITC staining was strongly revealed along the otherwise intact nuclear periphery (n, o) whereas it was depleted from cell surface (d, e). In marked contrast, the presence of STS conferred resistance against the acantholytic affects of PV serum (c), as cell morphology was comparable to controls (a). Panels a-e, anti-Dsg3 staining (FITC); panels f-j, nuclear staining (DAPI); panels k-o, merged images of Dsg3 extracellular domain and nuclei. Note that samples were processed simultaneously and photographic procedures held constant.

All mice receiving PV serum, but not control serum, developed skin blisters approximately 24 hours after a single injection. The blisters resulted from suprabasilar acantholysis, as revealed by histological examination (Figure 2, *normal serum and PV serum*).

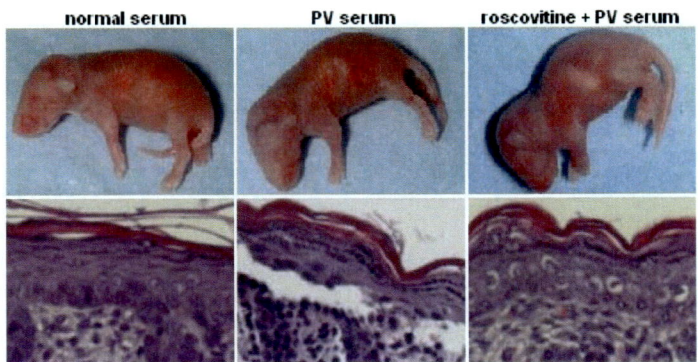

Figure 2. Central role for CDK2 in pemphigus vulgaris (PV). In neonatal mice injected with PV sera, pre-treatment with roscoivitine (100 µg/g body weight) prevents blister formation both clinically and histologically.

The passive transfer study was carried out in the presence of roscovitine, a well known inhibitor of cdk2 activity (33). 100 µg roscovitine per g of body weight dissolved in 20 µl PBS (n=6) or 20µl PBS as a control (n=6, not shown) were administered intraperitoneally 2 h before the i.p. injection of different PV sera. Remarkably, under our experimental conditions, none of mice (n=6) pre-treated with roscovitine developed any skin lesion, both clinically and histologically (Figure 2. *roscovitine pre-treatment followed by PV serum*) within 24 h after i.p. injection with PV sera (n=4).

Cdk2 Partially Modulates Gene Expression by PV Sera in Mouse Skin by DNA Microarray

To elucidate the molecular mechanism of roscovitine action on mice treated with PV serum, cRNA was generated from a pool of different mRNA isolated from skin samples of mice (n=6). In this experiment we have decided to use PV serum. In pilot array study on keratinocytes, we determined that PV serum induced important changes in transcription of the genes coding for one and the same proteins with known biological functions involved in PV disease (39). Arrays contained 14,000 well-characterized mouse genes (22,000 total genes comprehensive of EST sequences) were used to measure effects of treatments of mice with PV serum *versus* normal serum (see also chapter 8), PV serum in presence of roscovitine *versus* PV serum and PV serum in presence of roscovitine *versus* normal serum. In this case we have considered only genes that have the threshold of 50 arbitrary detection unit and absolute fold change value greater or equal than 2 have been included in the complete lists of genes (upon request as supplementary data). Overall, PV serum decreased transcription of 1114 genes and increased transcription of 349 genes, as detailed in chapter 8. *Roscovitine* modified the gene expression profile in the presence of PV serum. Compared with the effect of PV serum alone, exposure to PV serum in presence of roscovitine showed up-regulation of 117 genes and down-regulation of 153 genes, using the same filter criteria adopted for the comparison of PV serum versus normal serum. Additionally, some genes down-regulated or up-regulated in the presence of PV serum alone were up-regulated or down-regulated respectively when treated with roscovitine (ie, plakophilin 3, jagged 2, and calpain 6) (Table 1, Figure 3). Importantly, the comparison of PV serum in presence of roscovitine with NS showed that the vast majority of genes differentially expressed in PV serum alone and in presence of roscovitine were not differently expressed. In addition, Table 2 shows a list of some genes down and up regulated in presence of PV serum and re-established expression of genes by roscovitine. The biological process ontology and KEGG pathway terms associated with the differentially expressed genes were examined using the online available DAVID bioinformatics database.

The reciprocal changes were observed in transcription of the genes coding for proteins with known biological functions as follows: 1) components of cell organization and structure (keratins, transglutaminase, and involucrin); 2) cells adhesion molecules (jagged 2, desmoplakin, bystin-like, reelin, and calpain 6); 3) regulators of cell cycle progression (cyclin-dependent kinase 8, cyclin D1, cyclin D2, and cyclin G associated kinase; 5) cell death (cyclin-dependent kinase inhibitor 1A (P21), Fas death domain-associated protein, and growth arrest specific 1); 6) defense response (CD93 antigen, and histocompatibility 2, D region); 7) immuno response (histocompatibility 2, D region locus 1, and Interferon activated gene 203).

As usual, to validate data obtained by microarray analysis, we performed PCR on several differentially expressed genes involved in cell communication pathways.

The levels of induction detected by RT-PCR were similar to those observed on the microarrays. (Figure 3).

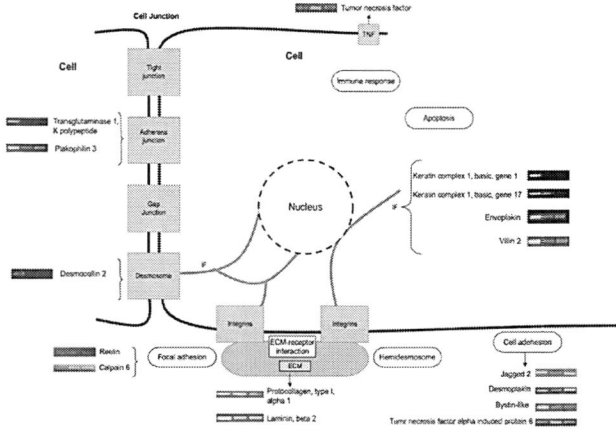

Figure 3. Pathway diagram (DAVID/KEGG database) showing genes involved in cell communication differentially regulated by PV serum with and without roscovitine treatment. The genes showed were confirmed by RT-PCR. For each amplification the first lane on the left is normal serum, the second lane is PV serum and third lane on the right is PV serum with roscovitine treatment. PV serum induced a significant variation in gene expression implicated in direct cell-cell contacts. Roscovitine treatment partially re-established the expression of these genes.

Table 1. Gene expression of samples treated with pemphigus vulgaris serum in presence of roscovitine *versus* pemphigus vulgaris serum (PVS/roscovitine *vs* PVS) and (PVS/roscovitine *vs* NS). The results are expressed as both the signal log ratio (SRL) and the direction of the change, i.e. an increase (I), a decrease (D). or no differential expression (NDE)

Representative Public ID	Gene title	Gene Ontology (Biological Process)	PVS + roscovitine *vs* PVS (SLR)	PVS + roscovitie *vs* NS (SLR)
D89901	keratin associated protein 6-3	Unknown	4.4 I	NDE

Table 1. (Continued)

Representative Public ID	Gene title	Gene Ontology (Biological Process)	PVS + roscovitine vs PVS (SLR)	PVS + roscovitie vs NS (SLR)
NM_054097	Phosphatidylinositol 4-phosphate 5 kinase, type II, gamma	Unknown	4.1I	NDE
NM_016879	keratin complex 2, basic, gene 18	Unknown	4.3I	2.7D
NM_009387	thymidine kinase 1	DNA replication	4.1I	NDE
NM_010666	keratin complex-1, acidic, gene C29	Cytoskeleton Organization And biogenesis	3.7I	3.7D
NM_025276	envoplakin	keratinization	3.7I	1.0D
BB283187	carnitine O octanoyltransferase	Lipid metabolism	3.6I	1.9D
NM_016705	kinesin family member 21A	Microtubule based process	3.4I	NDE
BC019374	glutamate-cysteine ligase, catalytic subunit	Glutathione biosynthesis	3.3I	1.7D
BC027245	Gamma aminobutyric acid (GABA-A) receptor, pi	transport	3.2I	NDE
NM_010659	keratin complex 1, acidic, gene 1	Cytoskeleton Organization and biogenesis	3.0I	5.5D
NM_010864	myosin Va	Cytoskeleton Organization And biogenesis	2.9I	1.3D
AK005226	calcium binding protein 39	Unknown	2.8I	NDE
BC025618	ATPase, Na+/K+ transporting, alpha 1 polypeptide	Transport	2.7I	1.6D

Representative Public ID	Gene title	Gene Ontology (Biological Process)	PVS + Roscovitine vs PVS (SLR)	PVS + roscovitie vs NS (SLR)
NM_134131	tumor necrosis factor, alpha-induced protein 8	Unknown	2.6I	NDE
BC024835	structure specific recognition protein 1	regulation of transcription, DNA dependent	2.3I	NDE
BM208103	Cytoskeleton associated protein 2	Unknown	2.4I	NDE
NM_022886	sciellin	Epidermis development	2.1I	NDE
NM_008631	metallothionein 4	Electron transport	2.0I	3.8D
AF083876	Epithelial membrane protein 2	Unknown	1.8I	1.9D
BG079188	bystin-like	cell adhesion	1.5I	1.0D
NM_012006	acyl-CoA thioesterase 1	long-chain fatty acid metabolism	1.5I	1.1D
AF296657	Ubiquitin conjugating enzyme E2G 2	Protein modification	1.4I	NDE
BM119387	villin 2	regulation of cell shape	1.3I	2.0D
NM_007991	fibrillarin	rRNA processing	1.3I	1.4D
NM_009983	cathepsin D	proteolysis	1.1I	1.1D
AK020708	glycoprotein, synaptic 21	Unknown	1.0I	2.3D

Table 1. (Continued)

Representative Public ID	Gene title	Gene Ontology (Biological Process)	PVS + Roscovitine vs PVS (SLR)	PVS + roscovitie vs NS (SLR)
X75650	keratin complex 1, acidic, gene 3	Cytoskeleton Organization and biogenesis	NDE	7.9D
AA727386	keratin associated protein 8-1	Unknown	NDE	5.9D
NM_009257	serine (or cysteine) peptidase inhibitor, clade B, member 5	Unknown	NDE	5.7D
NM_011060	peptidyl arginine deiminase, type III	Protein modification	NDE	5.2D
AF087470	S100 calcium binding protein A3	Electron transport	NDE	4.0D
X00246	Histocompatibility 2, D region locus 1	Immune response	NDE	3.6D
BC004663	Desmocollin 2	cell adhesion	NDE	NDE
AI506986	gasdermin 1	Unknown	NDE	3.7D
BC026422	transglutaminase 1, K polypeptide	Protein modification	NDE	NDE
BC026051	laminin, beta 2	Electron transport	NDE	NDE
BB006219	tyrosinase-related protein 1	Melanin Biosynthesis from tyrosine	NDE	3.0D
M98547	receptor-like tyrosine kinase	protein amino acid phosphorylaton	NDE	4.1D
BI410170	ribonuclease T2	Unknown	NDE	2.9D
AA798563	keratin complex 1, acidic, gene 17	Cellular morphogenesis	NDE	2.5D
AW475993	plakophilin 3	cell adhesion	NDE	2.0D
AV241768	tumor-associated calcium signal transducer 2	Defense response	NDE	NDE
BC014783	Proteasome (prosome, macropain) subunit, beta type 3	Ubiquitin Dependent Protein catabolism	NDE	1.6D

Representative Public ID	Gene title	Gene Ontology (Biological Process)	PVS + Roscovitine vs PVS (SLR)	PVS + roscovitine vs NS (SLR)
NM_009140	chemokine (C-X-C motif) ligand 2	chemotaxis	1.0D	3.4I
NM_010516	cysteine rich protein 61	regulation of cell growth	1.5D	1.7I
NM_007429	angiotensin II receptor, type 2	Angiotensin Mediated Vasodilation During regulation of blood pressure	1.5D	1.8I
BB241535	suppressor of cytokine signaling 3	regulation of cell growth	1.4D	1.3I
AV026617	FBJ osteosarcoma oncogene	regulation of progression through cell cycle	1.1D	2.8I
Representativ Public ID	Gene title	Gene Ontology (Biological Process)	PVS + Roscovitine vs PVS (SLR)	PVS + roscovitine vs NS (SLR)
BB238025	ZXD family zinc finger C	Unknown	1.6D	3.5I
NM_009398	tumor necrosis factor alpha induced protein 6	cell adhesion	NDE	
NM_011993	Dihydropyrimidinae-like 4	Unknown	NDE	NDE
AY027660	hornerin	development	NDE	5.1I
BB225239	Interleukin 10 receptor, alpha	cell surface receptor linked signal transduction	NDE	NDE
BC026555	kallikrein B, plasma 1	proteolysis	NDE	NDE
NM_011261	reelin	Cellular Morphogenesis During differentiation	NDE	NDE
AI747133	calpain 6	Cellular Morphogenesis During differentiation	NFD	2.2I
BI794771	procollagen, type I, alpha 1	Phosphate transport	NDE	2.0I

Discussion

As a final step of these experimental sections, we reported that pharmacological inhibition of cdk2 by roscovitine prevented blister formation in the neonatal mouse model of the disease. Thus, cdk2 is essential for PV blistering *in vivo*. Furthermore, we showed by microarray analysis that PV sera-induced changes in gene expression and regulatory events is regulated, at least in part, by cdk2 in mouse skin.

Mouse injected with roscovitine, an inhibitor of cdk2, before receiving PV serum did not develop any skin lesion. This finding provides strong evidence that activation of cdk2-mediated signaling is a crucial event of the acantholytic process *in vivo* and that pharmacological block of cdk2 can prevent PV skin blistering in mice. Recent studies report that also p38MAPK and c-Myc may be pharmacologically targeted in order to inhibit PV-like blistering [87,88]. We do not actually know whether PG, p38MAPK, cdk2, and c-Myc are members of the same 'acantholytic cascade' or whether they represent effectors of different signal transduction leading independently to cell-cell detachment. However, results reported here revealed cdk2 to be a key protein in PV pathogenesis and opened new perspectives toward a more targeted therapy of the disease. Indeed, the current treatment of PV patients is based on the non-selective use of steroideal and immunosuppressive agents [1]. Our findings implicate that the molecular effects of PV could be targeted by using selective cdk2 inhibitors. However, safety approach of such inhibitors in humans must be properly addressed.

The microarray that we designed on mice skin treated with PV serum was intended to evaluate the expression of know and unknown genes by comparing the gene expression with the response to roscovitine. PV serum seems to reduce the adhesion strength among keratinocytes by acting on the transcriptional level through the down-regulation of desmosomal proteins. It is worth of note that these 'slower' changes in gene regulation were abrogated by roscovitine, thus showing that cdk2 is crucial in orchestrating intracellular signalling which impair desmosome adhesion strength in pemphigus thus resulting in acantholysis. To date, further experiments are undergoing in our laboratories to assess more precise regulatory framework of cluster genes involved in in acantholysis during PV.

Concluding Remarks

In conclusion, the results presented here demonstrate that acantholysis can be prevented by pharmacological inhibition of cdk2. Our studies demonstrate how integration of molecular bioscience and systems levels analysis can be applied in human disease. Specifically, our results open new avenues for a safe non-steroideal treatment of pemphigus.

Acknowledgments

A big thanks goes to all my past and current collaborators, who contributed to the work published:

Alessandro Lanza
Fernando Gombos
Felice Femiano
Claudio Napoli
Stephen S. Prime

References

[1] Bystryn JC, Rudolph JL. Pemphigus. Lancet 2005; 366:61-73.
[2] Amagai M. Autoimmunity against desmosomal cadherins in pemphigus. J Dermatol Sci 1999; 20:92-102.
[3] Wolff K, Schreiner E. Ultrastructural localization of pemphigus autoantibodies within the epidermis. Nature 1971; 229:59-61.
[4] Patel HP, Diaz LA, Anhalt GJ, Labib RS, Takahashi Y. Demonstration of pemphigus antibodies on the cell surface of murine epidermal cell monolayers and their internalization. J Invest Dermatol 1984; 83:409-15.
[5] Shimizu A, Ishiko A, Ota T, et al. Ultrastructural changes in mice actively producing antibodies to desmoglein 3 parallel those in patients with pemphigus vulgaris. Arch Dermatol Res 2002; 294:318-23.
[6] Mascarò JM, Espana A, Liu Z, et al. Mechanisms of acantholysis in pemphigus vulgaris: role of IgG valence. Clin Imm Immunopat 1997; 85:90-6.
[7] Harman KE, Seed PT, Gratian MJ, Bhogal BS, Challacombe SJ, Black MM. The severity of cutaneous and oral pemphigus is related to desmoglein 1 and 3 antibody levels. Br J Dermatol 2001; 144:775-80.
[8] Nguyen VT, Ndoye A, Shultz LD, Pittelkow MR, Grando SA. Antibodies against keratinocyte antigens other than desmogleins 1 and 3 can induce pemphigus vulgaris-like lesions. J Clin Invest 2000; 106:1467-79.
[9] Cirillo N, Gombos F, Lanza A. Pemphigus vulgaris immunoglobulin G can recognize a 130,000 MW antigen other than desmoglein 3 on peripheral blood mononuclear cell surface. Immunology 2007; 121:377-82.
[10] Amagai M, Klaus-Kovtun V, Stanley JR. Autoantibodies against a novel epithelial cadherin in pemphigus vulgaris, a disease of cell adhesion. Cell 1991; 67:869-77.

[11] Ding X, Diaz LA, Fairley JA, Giudice GJ, Liu Z. The anti-desmoglein 1 autoantibodies in pemphigus vulgaris sera are pathogenic. J Invest Dermatol 1999; 112:739-43.
[12] Stanley JR, Year M, Hawley Nelson P, Katz SI. Pemphigus antibodies identify a cell surface glycoprotein synthesized by human and mouse keratinocytes. J Clin Invest. 1982; 70:281-8.
[13] Hashimoto T, Ogawa MM, Konohana A, Nishikawa T. Detection of pemphigus vulgaris and pemphigus foliaceus antigens by immunoblot analysis using different antigen sources. J Invest Dermatol 1990; 94:327-31.
[14] Getsios S, Huen AC, Green KJ. Working out the strength and flexibility of desmosomes. Nat Rev Mol Cell Biol 2004; 5: 271-81.
[15] Amagai M, Karpati S, Prussick R, Klaus-Kovtun V, Stanley JR. Autoantibodies against the amino-terminal cadherin-like binding domain of pemphigus vulgaris antigen are pathogenic. J Clin Invest 1992; 90:919-26.
[16] Futei Y, Amagai M, Sekiguchi M, Nishifuji K, Fujii Y, Nishikawa T. Use of domain-swapped molecules for conformational epitope mapping of desmoglein 3 in pemphigus vulgaris. J Invest Dermatol 2000; 115:829-34.
[17] Sekiguchi M, Futei Y, Fujii Y, Iwasaki T, Nishikawa T, Amagai M. Dominant autoimmune epitopes recognized by pemphigus antibodies map to the N-terminal adhesive region of desmogleins. J Immunol 2001; 167:5439-48.
[18] Tsunoda K, Ota T, Aoki M, et al. Induction of pemphigus phenotype by a mouse monoclonal antibody against the amino-terminal adhesive interface of desmoglein 3. J Immunol 2003; 170:2170-8.
[19] Nagasaka T, Nishifuji K, Ota T, Whittock NV, Amagai M. Defining the pathogenic involvement of desmoglein 4 in pemphigus and staphylococcal scaled skin syndrome. J Clin Invest 2004; 114:1484-92.
[20] Mahoney MG, Wang ZH, Rothenberger K, Koch PJ, Amagai M, Stanley JR. Explanation for the clinical and microscopic localization of lesions in pemphigus foliaceus and vulgaris. J Clin Invest 1999; 103:461-8.
[21] Korman NJ, Eyre RW, Klaus-Kovtun V, Stanley JR. Demonstration of an adhering-junction molecule (plakoglobin) in the autoantigens of pemphigus foliaceus and pemphigus vulgaris. N Engl J Med 1989; 321:631-5.
[22] Dmochowski M, Hashimoto T, Garrod DR, Nishikawa T. Desmocollins I and II are recognized by certain sera from patients with various types

of pemphigus particularly Brazilian pemphigus foliaceus. J Invest Dermatol 1993; 100:380-4.
[23] Mimouni D, Foedinger D, Kouba DJ, et al. Mucosal dominant pemphigus vulgaris with anti-desmoplakin autoantibodies. J Am Acad Dermatol 2004; 51:62-67.
[24] Schumann H, Baetge J, Tasanen K, et al. The shed ectodomain of collagen XVII/BP180 is targeted by autoantibodies in different blistering skin diseases. Am J Pathol 2000; 156:685-95.
[25] Nguyen VT, Ndoye A, Grando SA. Novel human □9 acetylcholine receptor regulating keratinocyte adhesion is targeted by pemphigus vulgaris autoimmunity. Am J Pathol 2000; 157:1377-91.
[26] Bastian BC, Nuss B, Romisch J, Kraus M, Brocker EB. Autoantibodies to annexins: A diagnostic marker for cutaneous disorders? J Dermatol Sci 1994; 8:194-202.
[27] Nguyen VA, Ndoye A, Grando SA. Pemphigus vulgaris antibody identifies pemphaxin, a novel keratinocyte annexin-like molecule binding acetylcholine. J Biol Chem 2000; 275:29466-76.
[28] Feliciani C, Toto P, Amerio P, et al. In vitro and in vivo expression of interleukin-1α and tumor necrosis factor-α mRNA in pemphigus vulgaris: interleukin-1α and tumor necrosis factor-α are involved in acantholysis. J Invest Dermatol 2000; 114:71-7.
[29] Feliciani C, Toto P, Wang B, Sauder DN, Amerio PL, Tulli A. Urokinase plasminogen activator mRNA is induced by IL-1α and TNF-α in in vitro acantholysis. Exp Dermatol 2003; 12:466-71.
[30] Lopez-Robles E, Avalos-Diaz E, Vega-Memije E, et al. TNF-α and IL-6 are mediators in the blistering process of pemphigus. Int J Dermatol 2001; 40:185-8.
[31] Bhol KC, Rojas AI, Khan IU, Ahmed AR. Presence of interleukin 10 in the serum and blister fluid of patients with pemphigus vulgaris and pemphigoid. Cytokine 2000; 12:1076-83.
[32] Eberhard Y, Burgos E, Gagliardi J, et al. Cytokine polymorphisms in patients with pemphigus. Arch Dermatol Res 2005; 296:309-13.
[33] Baroni A, Buommino E, Paoletti I, Orlando M, Ruocco E, Ruocco V. Pemphigus serum and captopril induce heat shock protein 70 and inducile nitric oxide synthase overexpression, triggering apoptosis in human keratinocytes. Br J Dermatol 2004; 150:1070-80.
[34] Pelacho B, Natal C, Espana A, Sanchez-Carpintero I, Iraburu MJ, Lopez-Zabalza MJ. Pemphigus vulgaris autoantibodies induce apoptosis in HaCaT keratinocytes. FEBS Lett 2004; 566:6-10.

[35] Wang X, Bregegere F, Frusic-Zlotkin M, Feinmesser M, Michel B, Milner Y. Possible apoptotic mechanism in epidermal cell acantholysis induced by pemphigus vulgaris autoimmunoglobulins. Apoptosis 2004; 9:131-43.
[36] Seishima M, Esaki C, Osada K, Mori S, Hashimoto T, Kitajima, Y. Pemphigus IgG, but not bullous pemphigoid IgG, causes a transient increase in intracellular calcium and inositol 1,4,5-triphosphate in DJM-1 cells, a squamous cell carcinoma line. J Invest Dermatol 1995; 104:33-7.
[37] Osada K, Seishima M, Kitajima Y. Pemphigus IgG activates and translocates protein kinase C from the cytosol to the particulate/cytoskeleton fractions in human keratinocytes. J Invest Dermatol 1997; 108:482-7.
[38] Berkowitz P, Hu P, Liu Z, et al. Desmosome signaling. Inhibition of p38MAPK prevents pemphigus vulgaris IgG-induced cytoskeleton reorganization. J Biol Chem 2005; 280, 23778-84.
[39] Wang X, Bregegere F, Soroka Y, Frusic-Zlotkin M, Milner Y. Replicative senescence enhances apoptosis induced by pemphigus autoimmune antibodies in human keratinocytes. FEBS Lett 2004; 567:281-6.
[40] Garrod DR, Merritt AJ, Nie Z. Desmosomal cadherins. Curr Opin Cell Biol 2002; 14:537-45.
[41] Seishima M, Satoh S, Nojiri M, Osada K, Kitajima Y. Pemphigus IgG induces expression of urokinase plasminogen activator receptor on the cell surface of cultured keratinocytes. J Invest Dermatol 1997; 109:650-5.
[42] Aoyama Y, Kitajima Y. Pemphigus vulgaris-IgG causes a rapid depletion of desmoglein 3 (Dsg3) from the Triton X-100 soluble pools, leading to the formation of Dsg3-depleted desmosomes in a human squamous carcinoma cell line, DJM-1 cells. J Invest Dermatol 1999; 112:67-71.
[43] Aoyama Y, Owada MK, Kitajima Y. A pathogenic autoantibody, pemphigus vulgaris-IgG, induces phosphorylation of desmoglein 3, and its dissociation from plakoglobin in cultured keratinocytes. Eur J Immunol 1999; 29:2233-40.
[44] Behrendt N, Ronne E, Dano K. The structure and function of the urokinase receptor, a membrane protein governing plasminogen activation on the cell surface. Biol Chem Hoppe Seyler 1995; 376:269-79.

[45] Schiltz JR, Michel B, Papay R. Appearance of "pemphigus acantholysis factor" in human skin cultured with pemphigus antibody. J Invest Dermatol 1979; 73:575-81.

[46] Hashimoto K, Shafran KM, Webber PS, Lazarus GS, Singer KH. Anti-cell surface pemphigus autoantibody stimulates plasminogen activator activity of human epidermal cells. J Exp Med 1983; 157:259-72.

[47] Romer J, Lund LR, Eriksen J, Pyke C, Kristensen P, Dano K. The receptor for urokinase-type plasminogen activator is expressed by keratinocytes at the leading edge during re-epithelialization of mouse skin wounds. J Invest Dermatol 1994; 102:519-22.

[48] Katsuta Y, Yoshida Y, Kawai E, Kohno Y, Kitamura K. Urokinase-type plasminogen activator is activated in stratum corneum after barrier disruption. J Dermatol Sci 2003; 32:55-7.

[49] Mahoney MG, Wang ZH, Stanley JR. Pemphigus vulgaris and pemphigus foliaceus antibodies are pathogenic in plasminogen activator knockout mice. J Invest Dermatol 1999; 113:22-5.

[50] Patel HP, Diaz LA, Anhalt GJ, Labib RS, Takahashi Y. Demonstration of pemphigus antibodies on the cell surface of murine epidermal cell monolayers and their internalization. J Invest Dermatol 1984; 83:409-15.

[51] Jones JCR, Yokoo KM, Goldman RD. Further analysis of pemphigus autoantibodies and their use in studies on the heterogeneity, structure and function of desmosomes. J Cell Biol 1986; 102:1109-17.

[52] Shirakata Y, Amagai M, Hanakawa Y, Nishikawa T, Hashimoto K. Lack of mucosal involvement in pemphigus foliaceus may be due to low expression of desmoglein 1. J Invest Dermatol 1998; 110:76-8.

[53] Amagai M, Tsunoda K, Zillikens D, Nagai T, Nishikawa T. The clinical phenotype of pemphigus is defined by the anti-desmoglein autoantibody profile. J Am Acad Dermatol 1999; 40:167-70.

[54] Ding X, Aoki V, Mascaró JM, Lopez-Swiderski A, Diaz LA, Fairley LA. Mucosal and mucocutaneous (generalized) pemphigus vulgaris show distinct autoantibody profiles. J Invest Dermatol 1997; 109:592-6.

[55] Payne AS, Hanakawa Y, Amagai M, Stanley JR. Desmosomes and disease: pemphigus and bullous impetigo. Curr Opin Cell Biol 2004; 16:536-43.

[56] Grando SA, Pittelkow MR, Shultz LD, Dmochowski M, Nguyen VT. Pemphigus: an unfolding story. J Invest Dermatol 2001; 117:990-5.

[57] Lanza A, Cirillo N, Femiano F, Gombos F. How does acantholysis occur in pemphigus vulgaris: a critical review. J Cutan Pathol 2006; 33:401-12.

[58] Arteaga LA, Prisayanh PS, Warren SJP, Liu Z, Diaz LA, Lin MS. A subset of pemphigus foliaceus patients exhibits pathogenic autoantibodies against both desmoglein-1 and desmoglein-3. J Invest Dermatol 2002; 118:806-11.

[59] Cirillo N, Santoro R, Lanza M, Annese P, Gombos F, Lanza A. Mucocutaneous pemphigus vulgaris carrying high-titre anti-desmoglein 1 antibodies with skin lesions resembling pemphigus erythematosus. Clin Exp Dermatol 2007; doi:10.1111/j.1365-2230.2007.02554.x

[60] Kricheli D, David M, Frusic-Zlotkin, et al. The distribution of pemphigus vulgaris-IgG subclasses and their reactivity with desmoglein 3 and 1 in pemphigus patients and their first-degree relatives. Br J Dermatol 2000; 143:337-42.

[61] Hacker MK, Janson M, Fairley JA, Lin MS. Isotypes and antigenic profiles of pemphigus foliaceus and pemphigus vulgaris autoantibodies. Clin Immunol 2002; 105:64-74.

[62] Ayatollahi M, Joubeh S, Mortazavi H, Jefferis R, Ghaderi A. IgG4 as the predominant autoantibody in sera from patients with active state of pemphigus vulgaris. J Eur Acad Dermatol Venereol 2004; 18:241-2.

[63] Spaeth S, Riechers R, Borradori L, Zillikens D, Budinger L, Hertl M. IgG, IgA and IgE autoantibodies against the ectodomain of desmoglein 3 in active pemphigus vulgaris. Br J Dermatol 2001; 144:1183-8.

[64] Ueki H, Kohda M, Nobutoh T, et al. Antidesmoglein autoantibodies in silicosis patients with no bullous diseases. Dermatology 2001; 202:16-21.

[65] Warren SJ, Lin MS, Giudice GJ, et al. The prevalence of antibodies against desmoglein 1 in endemic pemphigus foliaceus in Brazil. Cooperative Group on Fogo Selvagem Research. N Engl J Med 2000; 343:23-30.

[66] Warren SJ, Arteaga LA, Rivitti EA. The role of subclass switching in the pathogenesis of endemic pemphigus. J Invest Dermatol 2003; 120:104-8.

[67] Caldelari R, de Bruin A, Baumann D, et al. A central role for the armadillo protein plakoglobin in the autoimmune disease pemphigus vulgaris. J Cell Biol 2001; 153:823-34.

[68] Iwatsuki K, Han GW, Fukuti R, et al. Internalization of constitutive desmogleins with the subsequent induction of desmoglein 2 in pemphigus lesions. Br J Dermat 1999; 140:35-43.

[69] Hanakawa Y, Matsuyoshi N, Stanley JR. Expression of desmoglein 1 compensates for genetic loss of desmoglein 3 in keratinocyte adhesion. J Invest Dermatol 2002; 119:27-31.

[70] Amagai M, Karpati S, Klaus-Kovtun V, Udey MC, Stanley JR. The extracellular domain of pemphigus vulgaris antigen (Desmoglein 3) mediates weak homophilic adhesion. J Invest Dermatol 1994; 102:402-8.

[71] Kowalczyk AP, Borgwardt IE, Green KJ. Analysis of desmosomal cadherin adhesive function and stoichiometry of the desmosomal cadherin:plakoglobin complex. J Invest Dermatol 1996; 107:293-300.

[72] Chitaev NA, Troyanovsky SM. Direct Ca2+-dependent heterophilic interaction between desmosomal cadherins, desmoglein and desmocollin, contributes to cell-cell adhesion. J Cell Biol 1997; 138:193-201.

[73] Koch PJ, Mahoney MG, Ishikawa H, et al. Targeted disruption of the pemphigus vulgaris antigen (desmoglein 3) gene causes loss of keratinocyte cell adhesion with a phenotype similar to pemphigus vulgaris. J Cell Biol 1997; 137:1091-102.

[74] Nguyen VT, Lee TX, Ndoye A, et al. The pathophysiological significance of nondesmoglein targets of pemphigus autoimmunity. Development of antibodies against keratinocyte cholinergic receptors in patients with pemphigus vulgaris and pemphigus foliaceus. Arch Dermatol 1998; 134:971-80.

[75] Grando SA, Horton RM, Mauro TM, Kist DA, Lee TX, Dahl MV. Activation of keratinocyte nicotinic cholinergic receptors stimulates calcium influx and enhances cell differentiation. J Invest Dermatol 1996; 107:412-8.

[76] Zia S, Ndoye A, Lee TX, Webber RJ, Grando SA. Receptor-mediated inhibition of keratinocyte migration by nicotine involves modulations of calcium influx and intracellular concentration. J Pharmacol Exp Ther 2000; 293:973-81.

[77] Williams CL, Hayes VY, Hummel AM, Tarara JE, Halsey TJ. Regulation of E cadherin-mediated adhesion by muscarinic acetylcholine receptors in small cell lung carcinoma. J Cell Biol 1993; 121:643-54.

[78] Conroy WG, Ogden LF, Berg DK. Cluster formation of α7-containing nicotinic receptors at interneuronal interfaces in cell culture. Neuropharmacology 2000; 39:2699-705.

[79] Nakayama H, Numakawa T, Ikeuchi H, Hatanaka H. Nicotine-induced phosphorylation of extracellular signal-regulated protein kinase and CREB in PC12h cells. J Neurochem 2001; 79:489-98.
[80] Dajas-Bailador FA, Soliakov L, Wonnacott S. Nicotine activates the extracellular signal-regulated kinase 1/2 via the α7 nicotinic acetylcholine receptor and protein kinase A, in SH-SY5Y cells and hippocampal neurones. J Neurochem 2002; 80:520-30.
[81] Grando SA. Autoimmunity to keratinocyte acetylcholine receptors in pemphigus. Dermatology 2000; 201:290-5.
[82] Nguyen VT, Arredondo J, Chernyavsky AI, Pittelkow MR, Kitajima Y, Grando SA. Pemphigus vulgaris acantholysis ameliorated by cholinergic agonists. Arch Dermatol 2004; 140:327-34.
[83] Grando SA. New approaches to the treatment of pemphigus. J Invest Dermatol Symp Proc 2004; 9:84-91.
[84] Szonyi M, Csermely P, Sziklai I. Acetylcholine-induced phosphorylation in isolated outer hair cells. Acta Otolaryngol 1999; 119:185-8.
[85] Vasioukhin V, Bauer C, Yin M, Fuchs E. Directed actin polymerization is the driving force for epithelial cell-cell adhesion. Cell 2000; 100:209-19.
[86] Esaki C, Seishima M, Yamada T, Osada K, Kitajima Y. Pharmacologic evidence for involvement of phospholipase C in pemphigus IgG-induced inositol 1,4,5-trisphosphate generation, intracellular calcium increase, and plasminogen activator secretion in DJM-1 cells, a squamous cell carcinoma line. J Invest Dermatol 1995; 105:329-33.
[87] Berkowitz P, Hu P, Warren S, Liu Z, Diaz LA, Rubenstein DS. p38MAPK inhibition prevents disease in pemphigus vulgaris mice. Proc Natl Acad Sci USA 2006; 103:12855-60.
[88] Williamson L, Raess NA, Caldelari R, et al. Pemphigus vulgaris identifies plakoglobin as key suppressor of c-Myc in the skin. EMBO J 2006; 25:3298-309.
[89] Waschke J, Spindler V, Bruggeman P, Zillikens D, Schmidt G, Drenckhahn D. Inhibition of Rho A activity causes pemphigus skin blistering. J Cell Biol 2006; 175:721-7.
[90] Kurzen H, Henrich C, Booken D, et al. Functional characterization of the epidermal cholinergic system in vitro. J Invest Dermatol 2006; 29:2458-72.
[91] Arredondo J, Chernyavsky AI, Karaouni A, Grando SA. Novel mechanisms of target cell death and survival and of therapeutic action of IVIg in pemphigus. Am J Pathol 2005; 167:1531–44.

[92] Liu X, Van Vleet T, Schnellmann RG. The role of calpain in oncotic cell death. Annu Rev Pharmacol Toxicol 2004; 44: 349–70.
[93] Grando SA. Biological functions of keratinocyte cholinergic receptors. J Investig Dermatol Symp Proc 1997; 2:41–8.
[94] Cirillo N, Femiano F, Gombos F, Lanza A. Metalloproteinase 9 is the outer executioner of desmoglein 3 in apoptotic keratinocytes. Oral Dis 2007; 13:341-5.
[95] Bystryn JC, Grando, SA. A novel explanation for acantholysis in pemphigus vulgaris: the basal cell shrinkage hypothesis. J Am Acad Dermatol 2006; 54:513-6.
[96] Ahmed AR, Wagner R, Khatri K, et al. Major histocompatibility complex haplotypes and class II genes in non-Jewish patients with Pemphigus vulgaris. Proc Natl Acad Sci USA 1991; 88:5056–60.
[97] Veldman CM, Gebhard KL, Uter W, et al. T cell recognition of desmoglein 3 peptides in patients with Pemphigus vulgaris and healthy individuals. J Immunol 2004; 172:3883–92.
[98] Anhalt GJ, Labib RS, Voorhees JJ, Beals TF, Diaz LA. Induction of pemphigus in neonatal mice by passive transfer of IgG from patients with the disease. N Engl J Med 1982; 306:1189-96.
[99] Yeh SW, Cavacini LA, Bhol KC, et al. Pathogenic human monoclonal antibody against desmoglein 3. Clin Immunol 2006; 120:68-75.
[100] Swanson DL, Dahl MV. Methylprednisolone inhibits pemphigus acantholysis in skin cultures. J Invest Dermatol 1983; 81:258-60.
[101] Nguyen V, Kadunce DP, Hendrix JD, Gammon WR, Zone JJ. Inhibition of neutrophil adherence to antibody by dapsone: a possible therapeutic mechanism of dapsone in the treatment of IgA dermatoses. J Invest Dermatol 1993; 100:349-55.
[102] Boukamp P, Petrussevska RT, Breitkreutz D, Hornung J, Markham A, Fusenig NE. Normal keratinization in a spontaneously immortalized aneuploid human keratinocyte cell line. J Cell Biol 1998; 106:761-71.
[103] Cirillo N, Gombos F, Lanza, A. Changes in desmoglein 1 expression and subcellular localization in cultured keratinocytes subjected to anti-desmoglein 1 pemphigus autoimmunity. J Cell Physiol 2007; 210:411-6.
[104] Lavker RM, Dong G, Zheng P, Murphy GF. Hairless micropig skin. A novel model for studies of cutaneous biology. Am J Pathol 1991; 138:687–97.
[105] Cirillo N, Femiano F, Gombos F, Lanza A. Serum from pemphigus vulgaris reduces desmoglein 3 half-life and perturbs its de novo

assembly to desmosomal sites in cultured keratinocytes. FEBS Lett 2006; 580:3276-81.
[106] Farb RM, Dykes R, Lazarus GS. Anti-epidermal-cellsurface Pemphigus antibody detaches viable epidermal cells from culture plates by activation of proteinase. Proc Natl. Acad Sci USA 1978; 75:459–63.
[107] Fan JL, Memar O, McCormick DJ, Prabhakar BS. BALB/c mice produce blister-causing antibodies upon immunization with a recombinant human desmoglein 3. J Immunol 163:6228–35.
[108] Cirillo N, Gombos F, Ruocco V, Lanza A. Searching for experimental models of Pemphigus vulgaris. Arch Dermatol Res 2007; 299:9-12.
[109] 109.Anhalt GJ, Till GO, Diaz LA, Labib RS, Patel HP, Eaglstein NF. Defining the role of complement in experimental Pemphigus vulgaris in mice. J Immunol 1986; 137:2835–40.
[110] Cirillo N, Lanza M, Rossiello L, Gombos F, Lanza A. Defining the involvement of proteinases in pemphigus vulgaris: evidence of matrix metalloproteinase-9 overexpression in experimental models of disease. J Cell Physiol 2007; 212:36-41.
[111] Puviani M, Marconi A, Cozzani E, Pincelli C. Fas ligand in Pemphigus sera induces keratinocyte apoptosis through the activation of caspase 8. J Invest Dermatol 2003; 120:164–7.
[112] Baroni A, Lanza A, Cirillo N, Brunetti G, Ruocco E, Ruocco V. Vesicular and bullous disorders: pemphigus. Dermatol Clin. 2007; 25:597-603.
[113] Lanza A, De Rosa A, Femiano F, et al. Internalization of non-clustered desmoglein 1 without depletion of desmoglein 1 from adhesion complexes in an experimental model of the autoimmune disease pemphigus foliaceus. Int J Immunopathol Pharmacol 2007; 20:355-61.
[114] Lanza A, Femiano F, De Rosa A, Cammarota M, Lanza M, Cirillo N. The N-terminal fraction of desmoglein 3 encompassing its immunodominant domain is present in human serum: implications for pemphigus vulgaris autoimmunity. Int J Immunopathol Pharmacol 2006; 19:399-407.
[115] Cirillo N, Femiano F, Dell'ermo A, Arnese P, Gombos F, Lanza A. A novel method to investigate pemphigus-induced keratinocyte dysmorphisms through living cell immunofluorescence microscopy. Virchows Arch 2007; 450:683-90.
[116] Cirillo N, Lanza M, De Rosa A, et al. The most widespread desmosomal cadherin, desmoglein 2, is a novel target of caspase 3-mediated apoptotic machinery. J Cell Biochem 2007; doi:10.1002/jcb.21431.

[117] Kowalewski C, Mackiewicz W, Schmitt D, Jablonska S, Haftek M. Cell–cell junctions in acantholytic diseases. Arch Dermatol Res 2001; 293:1–11.
[118] Waschke J, Bruggeman P, BaumgartnerW, Zillikens D, Drenckhahn D. Pemphigus foliaceus IgG causes dissociation of desmoglein 1-containing junctions without blocking desmoglein 1 transinteraction. J Clin Invest 2005; 115:3157–65.
[119] Yamamoto Y, Aoyama Y, Shu E, Tsunoda K, Amagai M, Kitajima Y. Anti-desmoglein 3 (Dsg3) monoclonal antibodies deplete desmosomes of Dsg3 and differ in their Dsg3-depleting activities related to pathogenicity. J Biol Chem 2007; 282:17866-76.
[120] Muller R, Svoboda V, Wenzel E, et al. IgG reactivity against non-conformational NH-terminal epitopes of the desmoglein 3 ectodomain relates to clinical activity and phenotype of pemphigus vulgaris. Exp Dermatol 2006; 15:606-14.
[121] Amagai M, Ishii K, Hashimoto T, Gamou S, Shimizu N, Nishikawa T. Conformational epitopes of pemphigus antigens (Dsg1 and Dsg3) are calcium dependent and glycosylation independent. J Invest Dermatol 1995; 105:243–7.
[122] Young P, Boussadia O, Halfter H, et al. E-cadherin controls adherens junctions in the epidermis and the renewal of hair follicles. EMBO J 2003; 22, 5723–33.
[123] Ioannides D, Hytiroglou P, Phelps RG, Bystryn JC. Regional variation in the expression of pemphigus foliaceus, pemphigus erythematosus, and pemphigus vulgaris antigens in human skin. J Invest Dermatol 1991; 96:159–61.
[124] Shimizu A, Ishiko A, Ota T, Tsunoda K, Amagai M, Nishikawa T. IgG binds to desmoglein 3 in desmosomes and causes a desmosomal split without keratin retraction in a pemphigus mouse model. J Invest Dermatol 2004; 122:1145–53.
[125] Ishii K, Harada R, Matsuo I, Shirakata Y, Hashimoto K, Amagai M. In vitro keratinocyte dissociation assay for evaluation of the pathogenicity of anti-desmoglein 3 IgG autoantibodies in pemphigus vulgaris. J Invest Dermatol 2005; 124:939-46.
[126] Lanza A, Cirillo N. Caspase-dependent cleavage of desmoglein 1 depends on the apoptotic stimulus. Br J Dermatol 2007; 156:400-2.
[127] Cirillo N, Lanza M, Femiano F, et al. If pemphigus vulgaris IgG are the cause of acantholysis, new IgG-independent mechanisms are the concause. J Cell Physiol 2007; 212:563-7.

[128] Grando SA. Pemphigus in the XXI century: new life to an old story. Autoimmunity 2006; 39:521-30.
[129] Cirillo N, Lanza A. Pemphigus acantholysis and steric hindrance: an unsolved equation. J Clin Invest 2006; http://www.jci.org/cgi/eletters/115/11/3157.
[130] Moncada B, Kettelsen S, Hernandez-Moctezuma JL, Ramirez F. Neonatal pemphigus vulgaris: Role of passively transferred pemphigus antibodies. Br J Dermatol 1982; 106:465-7.
[131] Mausacchio A, Hardwick KG. The spindle checkpoint: structural insight into dynamic signalling. Nat Rev Mol Cell Biol 2002; 3:731-41.
[132] Garcia JF, Camacho FI, Morente M, et al. Spanish Hodgkin Lymphoma Study Group. Hodgkin and Reed-Sternberg cells harbor alterations in the major tumor suppressor pathways and cell-cycle checkpoints: analyses using tissue microarrays. Blood 2003; 101:681-9.
[133] Olvera M, Harris S, Amezuca CA, et al. Immunohistochemical expression of cell cycle proteins E2F-1, Cdk2, Cyclin E, p27(Kip), and Ki-67 in normal placenta and gestational trophoblastic disease. Mod Pathol 2001; 14:1036-42.
[134] Harwell RM, Mull BB, Porter DC, Keyomarsi K. Activation of cyclin-dependent kinase 2 by full length and low molecular weight forms of cyclin E in breast cancer cells. J Biol Chem 2004; 279:12695-705.
[135] Nguyen VT, Arredondo J, Chernyavsky AI, Kitajima Y, Pittelkow M, Grando SA. Pemphigus vulgaris IgG and methylprednisolone exhibit reciprocal effects on keratinocytes. J Biol Chem 2004; 279:2135-46.
[136] Ahmed AR, Spigelman Z, Cavacini LA, Posner MR. Treatment of pemphigus vulgaris with rituximab and intravenous immune globulin. N Engl J Med 2006; 355:1772-9.
[137] Schmidt E, Seitz CS, Benoit S, Brocker EB, Goebeler M. Rituximab in autoimmune bullous diseases: mixed responses and adverse effects. Br J Dermatol 2007; 156:352-6.
[138] Kaldis P, Aleem E. Cell cycle sibling rivalry: Cdc2 vs. Cdk2. Cell Cycle 2005; 4:1491-4.
[139] Dobrev H, Popova L, Vlashev D. Proteinase inhibitors and pemphigus vulgaris. An in vitro and in vivo study. Arch Dermatol Res 1996; 288:648-55.
[140] Johnson JL, George SJ, Newby AC, Jackson CL. Divergent effects of matrix metalloproteinases 3, 7, 9, and 12 on atherosclerotic plaque stability in mouse brachiocephalic arteries. Proc Natl Acad Sci U S A 2005; 102:15575-80.

[141] Weiske J, Schoneberg T, Schroder W, Hatzfeld M, Tauber R, Huber O. The fate of desmosomal proteins in apoptotic cells. J Biol Chem 2001; 276:41175-81.
[142] Jacobson MD, Weil M, Raff MC. Role of Ced-3/ICEfamily proteases in staurosporine-induced programmed cell death. J Cell Biol 1996; 133:1041–51.
[143] Dusek RL, Getsios S, Chen F, et al. The differentiation-dependent desmosomal cadherin desmoglein 1 is a novel caspase-3 target that regulates apoptosis in keratinocytes. J Biol Chem 2006; 281:3614-24.
[144] Steinhusen U, Weiske J, Badock V, Tauber R, Bommert K, Huber O. Cleavage and shedding of E-cadherin after induction of apoptosis. J Biol Chem 2001; 276:4972-80.
[145] Grando SA, Glukhen'kii BT, Kostromin AP, Boiko I, Kutsenko NS, Korostash TA. The role of kallikrein-kinin system components in the pathogenesis of bullous skin lesions in pemphigus and pemphigoid. Vopr Med Khim 1990; 36:23–7.
[146] Rosatelli TB, Rosolino AM, Dellalibera-Joviliano R, Reis ML, Donadi EA. increased activity of plasma and tissue kallikreins, plasmakininase II and salivary kallikrein in pemphigus foliaceus (fogo selvagem). Br J Dermatol 2005; 152:650–7.
[147] Schaefer BM, Jaeger C, Kramer MD. Plasminogen activator system in pemphigus vulgaris. Br J Dermatol 1996; 135:726–32.
[148] Liu Z, Li N, Diaz LA, Shipley JM, Senior RM, Werb Z. Synergy between a plasminogen cascade and MMP-9 in autoimmune disease. J Clin Invest 2005; 115:879–87.
[149] Cirillo N, Dell'Ermo A, Gombos F, Lanza A. The specific proteolysis hypothesis of pemphigus: does the song remain the same? Med Hypotheses 2007; doi:10.1016/j.mehy.2006.12.067
[150] Singh NJ, Schwartz RH. The strength of persistent antigenic stimulation modulates adaptive tolerance in peripheral CD4+ T cells. J Exp Med 2003; 198:1107-17.
[151] Allen E, Yu QC, Fuchs E. Mice expressing a mutant desmosomal cadherin exhibit abnormalities in desmosomes, proliferation, and epidermal differentiation. J Cell Biol 1996; 133:1367–82.
[152] Dennis G Jr, Sherman BT, Hosack DA, et al. DAVID: Database for Annotation, Visualization, and Integrated Discovery. Genome Biol 2003; 4:P3.
[153] Gu LH, Coulombe PA. Keratin function in skin epithelia: a broadening palette with surprising a shades. Curr Opin Cell Biol 2007; 19:13-23.

[154] Coulombe PA, Omary MB. Hard and soft priciples defining the structure, function and regulation of keratin intermediate filaments. Curr Opin Cell Biol 2002; 14:110-22.
[155] Fuchs E, Cleveland DW. A structural scaffolding of intermediate filaments in health and disease. Science 1988; 279:514-19.
[156] Huber O. Structure and function of desmosomal proteins and their role in development and disease. Cell Mol Life Sci 2007; 60:1872-90.
[157] Chernyavsky AI, Arredondo J, Kitajima Y, Sato-Nagai M, Grando SA. Desmoglein versus non-desmoglein signaling in pemphigus acantholysis: characterization of novel signaling pathways downstream of pemphigus vulgaris antigens. J Biol Chem 2007; 282:13804-1Bystryn JC, Rudolph JL. Pemphigus. *Lancet* 2005; 366:61-73.
[158] Grando SA, Bystryn JC, Chernyavsky AI, Frusić-Zlotkin M, Gniadecki R, Lotti R, Milner Y, Pittelkow MR, Pincelli C.Apoptolysis: a novel mechanism of skin blistering in pemphigus vulgaris linking the apoptotic pathways to basal cell shrinkage and suprabasal acantholysis. *Exp Dermatol* 2009; 18:764-70.
[159] Kalish RS. Pemphigus vulgaris: the other half of the story. *J Clin Invest* 2000; 106:1433-5.
[160] Lanza A, Lanza M, Santoro R, Soro V, Prime SS, Cirillo N. Deregulation of PERK in the autoimmune disease pemphigus vulgaris occurs via IgG-independent mechanisms. *Br J Dermatol* 2011; 164:336-43.

Index

A

access, 11, 126
acetic acid, 98, 114
acetone, 81
acetylcholine, 1, 5, 7, 13, 15, 47, 157, 161, 162
acid, 81, 131, 132, 134, 135, 136, 146, 147, 148
acidic, 134, 135, 136, 146, 148
adhesion, 1, 2, 4, 5, 7, 9, 11, 12, 13, 14, 15, 16, 18, 20, 22, 32, 33, 34, 37, 38, 43, 44, 45, 46, 49, 50, 55, 56, 57, 59, 63, 67, 68, 69, 72, 73, 77, 78, 79, 88, 89, 90, 92, 95, 96, 107, 108, 111, 114, 116, 117, 121, 122, 123, 124, 127, 128, 129, 130, 131, 132, 133, 135, 136, 137, 138, 139, 140, 144, 147, 148, 149, 150, 155, 157, 161, 162, 164
adhesion strength, 63, 73, 77, 89, 90, 124, 139, 150
adhesions, 15
adhesive properties, 19
adverse effects, 109, 166
agonist, 14
algorithm, 126
American Heart Association, 25, 124
amino, 5, 32, 51, 80, 131, 132, 136, 148, 156
amino acid, 5, 32, 80

amino acids, 32, 80
ammonium, 81
anchorage, 74
anchoring, 2, 38
aneuploid, 163
angiogenesis, 131
angiotensin II, 136, 149
annotation, 126
antagonism, 15
antibody, 2, 6, 7, 11, 15, 22, 23, 25, 32, 37, 40, 43, 45, 46, 47, 53, 56, 58, 60, 62, 63, 65, 66, 67, 68, 73, 79, 81, 83, 84, 85, 87, 94, 106, 112, 118, 142, 155, 157, 159, 163, 164
anticholinergic, 15, 18
antigen, 5, 14, 15, 23, 27, 28, 33, 37, 46, 53, 63, 77, 78, 81, 83, 84, 85, 86, 93, 94, 122, 127, 129, 132, 138, 144, 155, 156, 161
antigenicity, 57
antigen-presenting cell, 15
APC, 15
apoptosis, 5, 6, 8, 16, 18, 33, 41, 46, 112, 118, 119, 120, 121, 127, 132, 133, 141, 157, 158, 164, 167
apoptosis pathways, 8
apoptotic pathways, 18, 119, 168
arginine, 135, 148
arteries, 166
atherosclerotic plaque, 166

atmosphere, 24, 39, 97, 125, 140
attachment, 15
autoantibodies, 1, 2, 5, 7, 8, 10, 11, 12, 13, 14, 20, 22, 23, 32, 38, 40, 46, 49, 50, 51, 55, 57, 59, 60, 67, 68, 77, 78, 79, 88, 96, 138, 155, 156, 157, 159, 160, 165
autoantigens, 1, 3, 13, 47, 93, 156
autoimmune diseases, 1, 2
autoimmunity, 7, 13, 20, 22, 32, 45, 49, 77, 86, 92, 93, 96, 121, 122, 138, 157, 161, 163, 164

B

base, 24
bicarbonate, 81
bioavailability, 32
bioinformatics, 128, 144
biopsy, 24, 25, 31, 46, 125
biosynthesis, 134, 146
blood, 77, 78, 80, 83, 86, 92, 93, 122, 130, 136, 149
blood pressure, 136, 149
body weight, 32, 127, 143
branching, 130
Brazil, 160
breast cancer, 166
buccal mucosa, 4
bullous pemphigoid, 120, 158

C

Ca^{2+}, 15, 56, 138, 161
calcium, 4, 5, 6, 16, 50, 52, 53, 56, 57, 78, 132, 133, 134, 135, 136, 138, 146, 148, 158, 161, 162, 165
cancer, 96
candidates, 114
carcinoma, 158, 161
caspases, 17, 18
catabolism, 131, 133, 136, 148
CDC, 127, 129
cDNA, 5, 125

cell biology, 1
cell culture, 1, 17, 27, 52, 79, 97, 108, 112, 161
cell cycle, 95, 96, 97, 99, 103, 104, 107, 108, 127, 128, 129, 130, 131, 132, 133, 139, 140, 144, 166
cell death, 15, 18, 82, 87, 112, 113, 129, 144, 162, 163, 167
cell differentiation, 161
cell fate, 45
cell line, 24, 30, 108, 158, 163
cell organization, 124, 127, 128, 144
cell signaling, 127, 138
cell surface, 7, 18, 30, 38, 45, 46, 55, 57, 58, 59, 62, 63, 68, 83, 86, 100, 106, 112, 131, 136, 142, 149, 155, 156, 158, 159
chemical, 112
chemiluminescence, 97
chemotaxis, 136, 149
chloroform, 98
classes, 1
classification, 2
cleavage, 18, 49, 61, 63, 72, 73, 78, 112, 118, 119, 121, 165
clinical examination, 26
clusters, 38, 45, 58, 59, 67, 86, 106, 122
CO_2, 24, 39, 97, 125, 140
coding, 123, 127, 128, 129, 143, 144
collagen, 5, 157
color, iv, 142
communication, 13, 123, 129, 144, 145
compensation, 6, 9, 10, 11, 50, 120, 121, 122
complement, 23, 32, 53, 164
complexity, 112
condensation, 113, 119, 141
Congress, iv
connective tissue, 24
consent, 23
constituents, 2
control group, 88
controversial, 6, 49, 74
controversies, 20
copyright, iv
Copyright, iv

correlation, 10, 11, 18
correlations, 9, 96, 104
corticosteroid therapy, 23
corticosteroids, 26
culture, 12, 17, 38, 39, 56, 61, 73, 111, 115, 118, 119, 122, 164
culture conditions, 38, 39, 56
culture medium, 111, 122
cysteine, 132, 133, 134, 135, 136, 146, 148, 149
cytokines, 5, 22, 33, 34, 75, 79, 94, 138
cytoplasm, 18, 28, 38, 42, 45, 73, 137
cytoskeleton, 15, 20, 26, 29, 37, 38, 40, 43, 44, 45, 46, 74, 95, 96, 129, 137, 158

D

damages, iv
database, 126, 128, 144, 145
defects, 67
deficit, 67, 122
degradation, 8, 13, 73, 108, 141
degradation rate, 108
Denmark, 25, 40, 52, 79
deposits, 25, 27, 40, 46
depth, 49, 102
deregulation, 124
dermatoses, 163
dermatosis, 3
dermis, 5, 11
desmosome, 7, 8, 12, 15, 38, 49, 50, 57, 68, 95, 96, 137, 138, 139, 150
detachment, 7, 8, 9, 15, 16, 22, 26, 29, 30, 37, 40, 43, 44, 45, 50, 61, 62, 63, 64, 72, 74, 86, 99, 100, 106, 107, 117, 119, 142, 150
detectable, 13, 41, 42, 44, 45, 60, 67, 86, 107, 115
detection, 13, 30, 126, 128, 144
detection techniques, 13
detergents, 46
diacylglycerol, 16
diffusion, 121
direct action, 88
discordance, 75

disease progression, 4, 50
diseases, 1, 2, 9, 95, 96, 109, 160, 165, 166
disintegrin, 121, 138
dissociation, 7, 15, 16, 64, 82, 88, 89, 91, 158, 165
distribution, 10, 47, 58, 59, 68, 87, 160
DNA, 1, 97, 119, 124, 126, 128, 130, 131, 133, 134, 143, 146, 147
DNA repair, 131
DNA sequencing, 124
donors, 23, 28, 80
down-regulation, 128, 138, 144, 150
drugs, 14

E

E-cadherin, 14, 46, 67, 107, 120, 121, 138, 165, 167
electron, 6, 130
electrophoresis, 23, 39, 98, 113, 125
ELISA, 1, 23, 97
encoding, 5, 137
endogenous synthesis, 41
enzymatic activity, 118
enzyme, 7, 91, 112, 135, 138, 147
enzyme-linked immunosorbent assay, 91
enzymes, 18, 121, 127
epidermis, vii, 1, 2, 7, 9, 10, 11, 13, 18, 22, 24, 33, 34, 42, 50, 77, 83, 86, 93, 94, 103, 115, 122, 138, 155, 165
epithelia, 10, 167
epithelial cells, 14, 38, 93, 137
epithelium, 121
equilibrium, 22, 33, 34, 67, 79, 111
EST, 126, 128, 144
evidence, 17, 22, 32, 33, 59, 66, 67, 68, 73, 75, 77, 78, 79, 91, 92, 94, 107, 109, 119, 120, 123, 137, 140, 150, 162, 164
evolution, 123, 139
excitation, 113
exclusion, 92
exercise, 79, 80
experimental condition, 29, 32, 65, 75, 107, 108, 115, 124, 128, 143

exposure, 18, 21, 30, 54, 55, 59, 62, 86, 89, 99, 101, 102, 108, 114, 116, 117, 121, 128, 144
extensor, 26, 27
external environment, 2
extraction, 41, 52, 75, 97, 100, 125, 140
extracts, 23, 27, 60, 83, 84, 85, 86, 92, 98, 113

F

FAD, 24, 25, 39, 82
fibroblast growth factor, 127
filament, 38, 137
films, 53, 97
filters, 52, 53, 79, 80, 83, 85, 98
fixation, 46
flaws, 11
flexibility, 156
fluid, 4, 157
fluorescence, 26, 28, 40, 42, 43, 45, 53, 55, 58, 59, 61, 62, 63, 64, 65, 75, 83, 85, 86, 91, 106, 116, 117
force, 15, 162
formaldehyde, 26, 40, 113
formation, 2, 5, 7, 8, 9, 11, 14, 15, 16, 22, 32, 34, 35, 42, 44, 49, 50, 55, 57, 61, 63, 72, 92, 93, 105, 106, 111, 112, 119, 120, 122, 132, 139, 143, 150, 158, 161
formula, 113
fragments, 41, 62, 72, 88, 90, 121
functional changes, 91
funding, 1

G

GABA, 134, 146
gamma globulin, 32, 94
gel, 23, 39, 81, 84, 85, 86, 98, 113, 114, 125
gene expression, 123, 124, 126, 128, 137, 138, 139, 144, 145, 150
gene regulation, 139, 150
genes, 123, 124, 126, 127, 128, 129, 137, 138, 143, 144, 145, 150, 163

genetic background, 22
genome, 124
glutamate, 134, 146
glycine, 80
glycosylation, 165
growth, 24, 39, 52, 57, 97, 125, 127, 129, 130, 131, 132, 133, 136, 140, 144, 149
growth arrest, 129, 130, 144
growth factor, 24, 39, 52, 127, 133
guanine, 127, 130

H

HaCaT cells, 24, 28, 29, 39, 42, 52, 58, 61, 63, 74, 80, 82, 88, 90, 98, 105, 115, 125, 140
hair, 162, 165
hair cells, 162
hair follicle, 165
half-life, 49, 52, 54, 55, 66, 67, 73, 163
haplotypes, 163
health, 168
heat shock protein, 157
heterogeneity, 159
histogram, 62, 66, 88, 102, 105
histological examination, 23, 127, 143
histology, 9, 27, 31
homeostasis, 67
host, 22
human, 1, 2, 7, 13, 21, 23, 24, 25, 28, 32, 34, 39, 40, 52, 79, 83, 85, 88, 97, 105, 108, 122, 124, 125, 126, 129, 151, 156, 157, 158, 159, 163, 164, 165
human body, 2
human genome, 124
hybridization, 124, 125
hypothesis, 5, 8, 9, 10, 11, 14, 15, 16, 19, 34, 67, 73, 75, 76, 111, 120, 163, 167

I

illumination, 98
image, 142
images, 26, 37, 40, 141, 142

immune function, 78
immunization, 164
immunofluorescence, 1, 2, 10, 23, 25, 26, 27, 28, 30, 37, 42, 43, 44, 45, 47, 54, 55, 57, 61, 64, 65, 73, 81, 82, 87, 93, 99, 100, 106, 111, 113, 116, 119, 141, 142, 164
immunoglobulin, 86, 88, 90, 91, 92, 155
immunoglobulins, 52, 91
immunohistochemistry, 1, 103
immunoprecipitation, 10, 13, 39, 53, 78, 81, 84, 98, 113
immunoreactivity, 39, 46, 53, 83
immunosuppressive agent, 109, 150
impetigo, 159
in vitro, 7, 9, 12, 14, 21, 22, 23, 24, 26, 28, 30, 31, 35, 37, 38, 40, 42, 45, 50, 60, 63, 68, 75, 80, 92, 94, 95, 97, 108, 111, 112, 116, 119, 121, 122, 123, 124, 137, 140, 141, 157, 162, 166
in vivo, 7, 14, 21, 22, 23, 31, 32, 34, 35, 46, 50, 67, 94, 95, 104, 107, 111, 112, 119, 120, 121, 123, 124, 137, 138, 140, 150, 157, 166
incubation time, 62, 63, 82
individuals, 3, 90, 163
inducer, 112
induction, 22, 78, 118, 122, 127, 129, 145, 160, 167
infection, 4
inhibition, 6, 15, 50, 119, 139, 150, 151, 161, 162
inhibitor, 18, 39, 99, 127, 129, 135, 141, 143, 144, 148, 150
initiation, 78
injury, iv
inositol, 16, 158, 162
integration, 67, 151
integrity, 1, 2, 20, 34, 38, 49, 67, 122, 125
intercellular contacts, 15, 38, 67, 87
interface, 51, 156
interference, 1, 9, 78
internalization, 9, 43, 46, 49, 58, 59, 68, 69, 73, 117, 155, 159
intervention, 94

involution, 20
ion transport, 133
issues, 21, 94
Italy, 98
IVIg, 162

K

K^+, 134, 146
keratin, 26, 29, 37, 38, 40, 43, 45, 46, 127, 133, 134, 135, 136, 137, 145, 146, 148, 165, 168
keratinocyte, 1, 2, 4, 5, 7, 9, 11, 12, 13, 14, 16, 18, 21, 22, 23, 24, 30, 32, 34, 35, 38, 39, 40, 44, 45, 46, 47, 52, 68, 75, 77, 78, 79, 81, 83, 84, 85, 86, 87, 92, 96, 97, 100, 101, 107, 108, 111, 112, 115, 116, 117, 119, 121, 122, 123, 131, 137, 138, 155, 157, 161, 162, 163, 164, 165
keratinocytes, 1, 2, 4, 6, 8, 12, 13, 15, 16, 18, 19, 22, 24, 26, 27, 28, 29, 30, 33, 34, 37, 38, 40, 41, 42, 44, 45, 46, 47, 49, 50, 54, 55, 56, 59, 60, 61, 63, 64, 65, 66, 68, 72, 73, 74, 75, 77, 78, 84, 86, 87, 88, 89, 90, 91, 92, 93, 94, 95, 96, 97, 99, 100, 101, 103, 104, 105, 106, 107, 108, 111, 112, 115, 116, 118, 119, 121, 122, 123, 124, 125, 126, 128, 129, 140, 141, 143, 150, 156, 157, 158, 159, 163, 164, 166, 167
kinase activity, 95, 96, 130, 141

L

labeling, 43
lead, 1, 2, 56
lesions, 4, 6, 12, 13, 21, 27, 31, 32, 33, 34, 94, 121, 122, 155, 156, 160, 167
ligand, 18, 136, 149, 164
light, 77, 92, 94, 120, 138
liver, 138
localization, 10, 45, 61, 85, 96, 112, 119, 155, 156, 163

M

mAb, 72, 74, 79
machinery, 68, 73, 100, 107, 164
magnitude, 126
majority, 42, 51, 116, 144
manipulation, 37, 63
mapping, 156
masking, 127
mass, 60, 72
materials, 31, 43, 64, 87, 99
matrix, 18, 33, 38, 88, 111, 114, 127, 164, 166
matrix metalloproteinase, 18, 33, 38, 111, 114, 164, 166
matter, iv
measurement, 97
mechanical stress, 2, 82, 88, 137
media, 39, 41, 42, 57, 82, 116
median, 61, 64
membranes, 2, 53, 84, 97, 98, 99, 113
Metabolic, 82, 88
metabolic intermediates, 75
metabolism, 26, 40, 78, 127, 129, 130, 133, 134, 135, 146, 147
metalloproteinase, 18
methanol, 25, 40, 98
methylation, 130
methylprednisolone, 166
MHC, 132
mice, 9, 12, 13, 14, 18, 21, 25, 31, 32, 33, 93, 94, 111, 112, 115, 120, 124, 125, 127, 128, 129, 137, 138, 142, 143, 150, 155, 159, 162, 163, 164
microarray technology, 124
microscope, 26, 40, 82, 126
microscopy, 30, 37, 38, 43, 44, 45, 47, 62, 63, 64, 65, 73, 81, 85, 87, 100, 106, 113, 116, 164
Microsoft, 54
migration, 7, 8, 13, 112, 161
mitochondria, 18

locus, 129, 135, 144, 148
lymph, 20

mitogen, 96, 132
mitosis, 96, 109
MMP, 33, 38, 111, 112, 113, 114, 115, 116, 117, 118, 119, 121, 122, 138, 167
MMP-2, 119
MMP-3, 114
MMP-9, 111, 112, 113, 114, 115, 116, 117, 118, 119, 121, 122, 167
MMPs, 112, 118, 119, 120, 121, 122
models, 1, 9, 21, 22, 23, 31, 32, 34, 35, 68, 78, 94, 111, 112, 124, 138, 164
modifications, 86, 96, 113
molecular mass, 13, 28, 49, 60, 72, 93, 94, 99, 108
molecular weight, 13, 85, 166
molecules, 2, 5, 13, 14, 15, 16, 18, 20, 22, 28, 33, 37, 47, 75, 78, 96, 107, 121, 123, 127, 128, 137, 138, 140, 144, 156
monoclonal antibody, 30, 51, 60, 61, 68, 79, 156, 163
monolayer, 24, 88
morphogenesis, 136, 148
morphology, 18, 43, 45, 46, 64, 77, 86, 87, 100, 108, 113, 119, 142
morphometric, 64, 75, 106, 107
motif, 136, 149
mRNA, 126, 128, 143, 157
mucosa, 1, 4, 10, 11, 24, 50
mucous membrane, 1, 2, 3, 11
mucous membranes, 1, 2, 11
mutant, 167
myosin, 134, 146

N

Na^+, 134, 146
NaCl, 39, 53, 80, 81, 98
National Institutes of Health, 25, 124
necrosis, 130, 147, 149, 157
neonates, 93
NH2, 51
nicotine, 161
nitric oxide, 157
nitric oxide synthase, 157
nitrogen, 125, 141

nuclei, 29, 87, 113, 142
nucleotides, 125
nucleus, 18, 26, 34, 37, 38, 40, 42, 44, 45, 73
null, 13, 93

O

oral lesion, 3, 26
organ, 2, 21, 23, 24, 30, 31, 32, 33, 34, 35, 40, 111, 115, 116, 119, 122, 123, 137
organelles, 2
overlap, 47
overlay, 142

P

palate, 4
parallel, 72, 86, 108, 109, 124, 155
participants, 23
pathogenesis, 1, 7, 8, 9, 14, 15, 20, 22, 31, 32, 33, 34, 75, 77, 78, 79, 93, 96, 108, 120, 150, 160, 167
pathophysiological, 2, 6, 7, 51, 92, 161
pathophysiology, 1, 20, 32, 34, 46, 61, 63, 78, 92, 93, 94, 96, 108, 123
pathways, 1, 13, 15, 16, 18, 19, 78, 107, 108, 121, 123, 129, 138, 140, 144, 166
PBMC, 77, 80, 81, 82, 83, 84, 85, 86, 92, 93, 94
PCR, 125, 126, 127, 129, 141, 144, 145
pemphigus, 1, 2, 3, 5, 6, 7, 9, 10, 11, 12, 13, 14, 15, 16, 18, 19, 20, 21, 22, 23, 26, 29, 31, 32, 33, 34, 35, 38, 44, 49, 50, 52, 56, 59, 67, 68, 72, 73, 74, 77, 79, 89, 90, 91, 92, 93, 97, 99, 112, 114, 120, 122, 129, 134, 139, 140, 143, 145, 150, 151, 155, 156,란157, 158, 159, 160, 161, 162, 163, 164, 165, 166, 167, 168
penicillin, 24, 39
peptidase, 131, 132, 133, 135, 148
peptide, 73, 122, 132
peptides, 163

periodontitis, 12, 22
peripheral blood, 14, 77, 122, 138, 155
peripheral blood mononuclear cell, 14, 77, 122, 138, 155
permeability, 18
permission, iv
pH, 7, 39, 53, 80, 81, 98, 114
phenol, 82
phenomenology, 93, 108
phenotype, 10, 11, 20, 27, 156, 159, 161, 165
phosphate, 24, 134, 146
phosphatidylcholine, 16
phosphorylation, 7, 13, 15, 89, 90, 95, 96, 99, 102, 107, 108, 124, 131, 132, 136, 140, 141, 158, 162
physiology, 1
placenta, 93, 166
plasma membrane, 18
plasminogen, 7, 8, 9, 112, 120, 138, 157, 158, 159, 162, 167
polyacrylamide, 23, 39, 81, 98, 113, 114
polymerization, 162
polymorphisms, 157
polypeptide, 130, 134, 135, 146, 148
polypropylene, 80
pools, 41, 74, 158
preparation, iv, 54, 125
principles, 1
probe, 126
proliferation, 13, 97, 112, 167
proline, 6
protease inhibitors, 52, 80
protection, 107
protein folding, 133
protein kinase C, 16, 96, 158
protein kinases, 96, 101, 103
protein synthesis, 52, 55, 141
proteinase, 7, 93, 111, 122, 164
proteins, 9, 14, 18, 28, 37, 38, 44, 45, 46, 60, 73, 81, 83, 95, 96, 98, 99, 108, 121, 122, 123, 127, 128, 129, 137, 144, 150, 166, 167, 168
proteolysis, 8, 73, 112, 120, 121, 122, 129, 132, 133, 135, 136, 138, 147, 149, 167

proteolytic enzyme, 7, 121
purification, 22, 23, 52, 81
PVM, 68
PVS, 129, 130, 131, 132, 133, 134, 135, 136, 137, 145, 146, 147, 148, 149

Q

quantification, 124

R

Rab, 132
reactions, 12
reactivity, 5, 61, 77, 85, 86, 92, 160, 165
reagents, 52, 79, 97
reasoning, 32
receptors, 1, 5, 7, 8, 13, 15, 22, 32, 47, 78, 138, 161, 162, 163
recognition, 12, 78, 134, 147, 163
recommendations, iv, 98
redistribution, 30, 43, 59, 68, 100, 142
regulatory framework, 150
relatives, 12, 22, 160
relevance, 14
remission, 22
repair, 9
replication, 134, 146
reproduction, 47
researchers, 34, 78
residues, 51, 72, 79
resistance, 108, 142
resolution, 43
respiration, 82
response, 15, 45, 50, 55, 59, 67, 68, 73, 75, 93, 116, 121, 124, 129, 135, 136, 137, 144, 148, 150
rights, iv
risk, 46
rituximab, 109, 166
RNA, 18, 95, 125, 133, 140, 141
RNAs, 125, 141
room temperature, 81
rules, 25, 124

S

safety, 109, 150
saturation, 46
secrete, 116
secretion, 7, 113, 116, 118, 119, 121, 122, 162
senescence, 158
sensitivity, 13
sequencing, 124
serine, 7, 8, 135, 148
serum, 2, 8, 9, 16, 19, 21, 23, 24, 25, 26, 27, 29, 30, 31, 32, 34, 38, 42, 44, 45, 46, 49, 50, 53, 54, 55, 56, 57, 58, 59, 60, 61, 62, 63, 64, 65, 66, 67, 68, 72, 73, 75, 78, 79, 80, 81, 85, 86, 87, 88, 89, 90, 91, 92, 93, 94, 95, 96, 97, 99, 100, 101, 102, 103, 104, 106, 107, 108, 111, 112, 113, 114, 115, 116, 117, 119, 121, 122, 123, 124, 126, 127, 128, 129, 134, 137, 138, 139, 140, 141, 142, 143, 145, 150, 157, 164
services, iv
shape, 14, 15, 37, 43, 44, 46, 47, 77, 79, 86, 87, 92, 100, 106, 107, 108, 135, 147
shock, 133
showing, 12, 13, 27, 55, 88, 102, 103, 139, 145, 150
sibling, 166
signal transduction, 7, 68, 150
signaling pathway, 8, 108, 168
signalling, 7, 13, 96, 139, 150, 166
signals, 1, 41, 54, 67, 73, 95, 111, 139
signs, 45, 86, 87, 100, 107, 141
silicosis, 12, 22, 160
siRNA, 80, 92, 98, 106, 107
skin, 1, 2, 3, 4, 7, 8, 12, 13, 14, 16, 21, 23, 24, 25, 26, 27, 30, 31, 32, 33, 34, 35, 40, 46, 95, 99, 103, 104, 105, 107, 108, 111, 115, 116, 119, 120, 122, 123, 124, 125, 127, 128, 137, 140, 143, 150, 156, 157, 159, 160, 162, 163, 165, 167, 168
skin diseases, 46, 157
sodium, 24, 39, 98, 113
solution, 24, 81, 82, 85, 98, 113, 114, 125

spectrophotometry, 125
speculation, 11
spindle, 166
squamous cell, 158, 162
squamous cell carcinoma, 158, 162
stability, 12, 38, 56, 67, 68, 96, 166
stable complexes, 67
starvation, 97
state, 38, 67, 99, 108, 140, 160
states, 14
sterile, 24
stimulus, 119, 121, 165
stoichiometry, 161
structural protein, 137
structure, 6, 19, 124, 127, 128, 134, 144, 147, 158, 159, 168
substrate, 23, 82, 88, 114, 119, 122
survival, 162
suspensions, 7
swelling, 18
syndrome, 131, 156
synergistic effect, 74
synthesis, 7, 9, 50, 59, 60, 97, 125

T

T cell, 121, 163, 167
target, 13, 33, 49, 89, 93, 122, 138, 162, 164, 167
techniques, 1, 22, 108
technologies, 124
technology, 124
telangiectasia, 131
therapeutic approaches, 109
therapy, 78, 94, 108, 123, 139, 150
time periods, 40
tissue, 2, 22, 26, 34, 38, 78, 93, 124, 166, 167
tissue homeostasis, 22
TNF, 5, 22, 79, 133, 138, 157
trafficking, 58, 68
transcription, 7, 127, 128, 129, 131, 133, 134, 143, 144, 147
transcripts, 124, 126, 141
transducer, 136, 148

transduction, 1, 15, 95, 96, 131, 132, 136, 139, 149
transfection, 99
transport, 130, 134, 135, 137, 138, 146, 147, 148, 149
treatment, 14, 20, 24, 30, 44, 45, 54, 55, 58, 59, 63, 66, 68, 73, 77, 86, 87, 90, 91, 92, 97, 100, 103, 106, 109, 112, 113, 128, 139, 143, 145, 150, 151, 162, 163
triggers, 19
trypsin, 7, 24, 57
tumor, 130, 134, 136, 147, 148, 149, 157, 166
tumor necrosis factor, 134, 136, 157
tyrosine, 135, 136, 148

U

UK, 26, 41
uniform, 88
urea, 39
urokinase, 129, 158, 159
USA, 162, 163, 164
UV, 98

V

valence, 155
validation, 9
vesicle, 38
visualization, 142

W

water, 98
wells, 53
western blot, 40, 42, 77, 84, 90, 111, 115
Western blot, 1, 23, 27, 28, 41, 49, 53, 54, 55, 60, 61, 62, 66, 72, 73, 75, 81, 83, 85, 90, 95, 98, 99, 101, 104, 105, 113, 114, 115, 119
worldwide, 124

Z

zinc, 112, 136, 149

SAFETY AND RISK IN SOCIETY

FEDERAL CYBERSECURITY PLANNING:

HUMAN CAPITAL AND RESEARCH AND DEVELOPMENT

KURK C. MOORE
AND
MARION D. TAYLOR
EDITORS

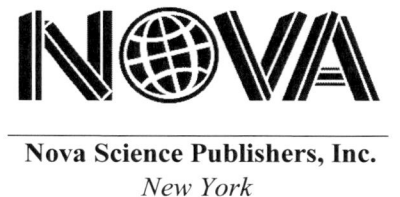

Nova Science Publishers, Inc.
New York

Copyright © 2012 by Nova Science Publishers, Inc.

All rights reserved. No part of this book may be reproduced, stored in a retrieval system or transmitted in any form or by any means: electronic, electrostatic, magnetic, tape, mechanical photocopying, recording or otherwise without the written permission of the Publisher.

For permission to use material from this book please contact us:
Telephone 631-231-7269; Fax 631-231-8175
Web Site: http://www.novapublishers.com

NOTICE TO THE READER

The Publisher has taken reasonable care in the preparation of this book, but makes no expressed or implied warranty of any kind and assumes no responsibility for any errors or omissions. No liability is assumed for incidental or consequential damages in connection with or arising out of information contained in this book. The Publisher shall not be liable for any special, consequential, or exemplary damages resulting, in whole or in part, from the readers' use of, or reliance upon, this material. Any parts of this book based on government reports are so indicated and copyright is claimed for those parts to the extent applicable to compilations of such works.

Independent verification should be sought for any data, advice or recommendations contained in this book. In addition, no responsibility is assumed by the publisher for any injury and/or damage to persons or property arising from any methods, products, instructions, ideas or otherwise contained in this publication.

This publication is designed to provide accurate and authoritative information with regard to the subject matter covered herein. It is sold with the clear understanding that the Publisher is not engaged in rendering legal or any other professional services. If legal or any other expert assistance is required, the services of a competent person should be sought. FROM A DECLARATION OF PARTICIPANTS JOINTLY ADOPTED BY A COMMITTEE OF THE AMERICAN BAR ASSOCIATION AND A COMMITTEE OF PUBLISHERS.

Additional color graphics may be available in the e-book version of this book.

Library of Congress Cataloging-in-Publication Data

ISBN 978-1-61942-769-3

Published by Nova Science Publishers, Inc. † New York